New Paradigms in Healthcare

AF147949

In the first two decades of this new millennium, the self-sufficiency of Evidence-Based Medicine (EBM) have begun to be questioned. The narrative version gradually assumed increasing importance as the need emerged to shift to more biologically, psychologically, socially, and existentially focused models. The terrible experience of the COVID pandemic truly revealed that EBM alone, while being a wonderful scientific philosophy and containing the physician's paternalistic approach, has its limitations: it often ignores both the patient's and physician's perspectives as persons, as human beings; it pays relentless attention to biological markers and not to the more personal, psychological, social, and anthropological ones, removing the emotions, thoughts, and desires of life, focusing on just the "measurable quality" of it.

Health Humanities, Medical Humanities and Narrative Medicine are arts intertwined with sciences that allow to broaden the mindset and approach of healthcare professionals. helping them to produce better care and more well-being.

Aim of this series is to collect "person-centered" contributions, as only a multidisciplinary and collaborative team can meet the challenge of combining the multiple aspects of human health, as well as the health of our planet, and of all the creatures that live on it, in a common effort to stop or reverse the enormous damage committed by humans during our anthropocentric era: a new paradigm of healthcare, education and learning to create a sustainable health system.

Elisabetta Pasini • Cinzia Trimboli

A Social Dreaming Experience at the Time of COVID 19

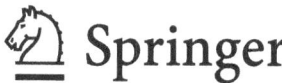

Springer

Elisabetta Pasini
Jungian Psychoanalyst
The Flying Carpet Studio, Milan - Zurich
C.G. Jung Institute for Analytical
Psychology
Milan, Italy

Cinzia Trimboli
Psychologist and Counselor
Order of Psychologists of Piedmont (OPP)
The Flying Carpet Studio
Turin, Italy

ISSN 2731-3247 ISSN 2731-3255 (electronic)
New Paradigms in Healthcare

ISBN 978-3-031-42500-4 ISBN 978-3-031-42498-4 (eBook)
https://doi.org/10.1007/978-3-031-42498-4

This Springer imprint is published by the registered company Springer Nature Switzerland AG
The registered company address is: Gewerbestrasse 11, 6330 Cham, Switzerland

Paper in this product is recyclable.

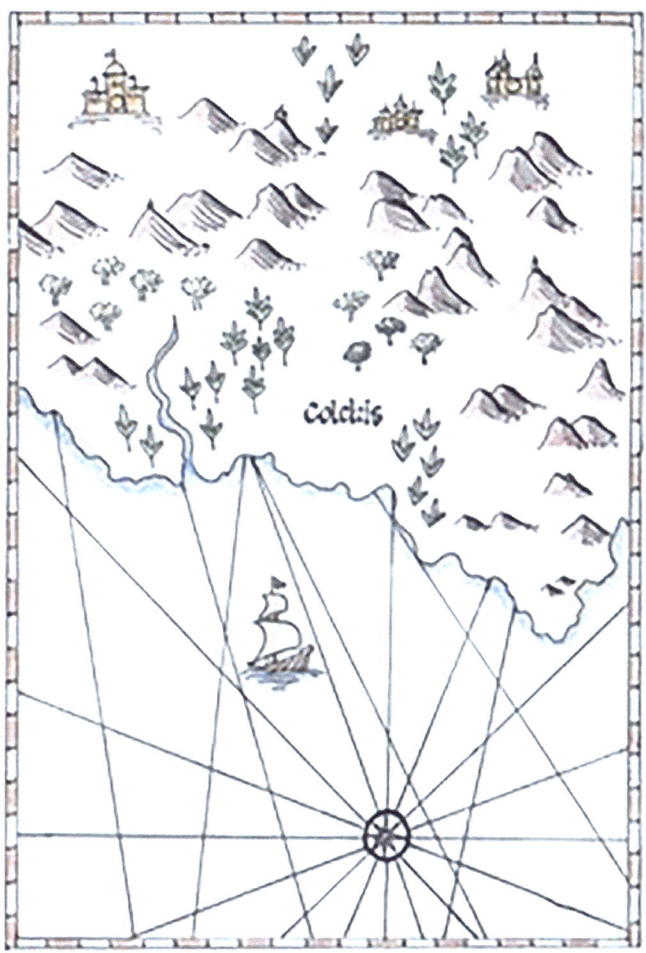

Original graphical illustration by the artist Roque Fucci

To the memory of my father, who taught me to love traveling, discovery, and movement. And to my husband and life companion, Ivan Mazzei, whose curious gaze toward the world is the most beautiful of the adventures I could have ever imagined to live.

Elisabetta Pasini

To my life partner, Marco Saracco, for his light-hearted spirit and openness to the world, for always being close to me, supporting me in difficulties and encouraging my passions. To my cat Beté, who has followed all the stages of this journey with an indolent and sleepy demeanor. Finally, this work is dedicated to my parents, who have strongly shaped the woman I am today.

Cinzia Trimboli

Foreword

Thinking the unthinkable

"*Today, we have a lot of contents but few containers to process the experience of change,*" Elisabetta Pasini and Cinzia Trimboli, dear friends and colleagues in many experiences of study and research, tell us. This is indeed the case. Even before the pandemic, there were many of us who found that the avalanche of events that the contemporary world has thrown at us—from the globalization of markets to the Twin Towers, from the global finance crisis to Daesh's online beheadings, from pushed digitization to migration phenomena, to COVID-19 and the Russian invasion of Ukraine—our ability to think, that is, to process events with thought, transforming them into experience, has been not to say nullified, but certainly greatly hampered, with the effect of generating and spreading confusion, bewilderment, and fears of various kinds: fear of the other, fear of the new, fear of the future....

Among the most nefarious effects of COVID-19 has undoubtedly been that it has crippled the habitual spaces and "natural" containers that, from the earliest moments of life, have structured our (inter)subjectivity: family, schoolmates, circle of friends, work colleagues, all removed and separated into isolated cells. At the same time, the great transformations of the surrounding world—networks and infosphere—extended to unimaginable, once unthinkable limits the relational container (I still recall Bion's statement concerning the fact that a group can be spoken of only when its members have the possibility of mutual visual relations).

Among the many merits I recognize in this book, I first and foremost grasp the point about the need to create new containers capable of restoring the capacity for thinking, a prerequisite to the possibility not only of understanding what is going on, but also and above all of transforming reality, that is, of making it—to put it in clinical terms—treatable. This is why I particularly agree with the passage in which, citing the "transformative thinking" theorized by Thomas Ogden, they quote his statement that "*This type of thinking always requires the minds of at least two people, since the isolated individual cannot radically change the fundamental categories of meaning with which he organizes his experience.*" The minds of at least two people. A concept that has always come to me to translate into "one never thinks alone."

In order to think about COVID-19, one must first recognize that *"the pandemic has pervasively affected the 'social bonds' that unite people."* An affirmation that I immediately brought back to the lesson of Renè Kaës when, in reference to man-made collective traumas (military dictatorships, political mass murders, the use of torture...), he highlighted how they attack the "structuring unconscious alliances" that ensure the formation of bonds, causing the catastrophic breakdown of the "metapsychic guarantors" of social life.

The traumatic situation, Kaës further asserts, produces a "community of denial" in which, analogous to the "psychic collapse" that for Winnicott characterizes the psychotic experience, a rupture in the ability to think and the short-circuiting of the ego's defense mechanisms, whether individual or institutional, opens up.

In search of containers—and here one cannot help but think of the great Bionian metaphor "container-contained"—in which to be able to reactivate the ability to think, the authors have found in Social Dreaming a resource that is not to say unhoped for but that is still in search of its full and recognized appreciation.

On Social Dreaming, as an approach and as a technique, I do not think it is for me to add to what the Authors present to us. In recent years, having experienced, still in the mid-1990s, on the one occasion when I met Gordon Lawrence, being taken back by him when I ventured to propose a comparison with other kinds of group experiences, I have had the opportunity to participate in a number of matrices and, in some cases, to try my hand at being the host. Thus, a little at a time, I matured and accepted the notion that the matrix, which in effect takes the form of a "group meeting," should not be considered a group experience, such as a T-group or a group-analysis session might be; instead, it is properly a research experience, one might even say a social experiment, in which the dreams not only do not belong to the individuals brought together to bring the matrix to life, but are not even of the group sharing them; that group, if anything, somehow and through some kind of process about the nature of which even the Authors continue to question, is able to attract and bring to the minds of the participants material that has a broader origin and scope, in time and space.

In this perspective—and here the research produced by the Authors proves particularly interesting—the function performed by the matrix of Social Dreaming is clarified by the dual meaning of the term: on the one hand, in a literal sense, the matrix is a kind of *"womb, incubator, an intermediate generative space in which something new can happen,"* a container, precisely; or, even more precisely, a *"habitat,"* a *"common frame"* that, said in the terms of a different theoretical model, acts as an intersubjective field created by the meeting of a group of people convened there; but, on the other hand, the matrix should also be understood as an *"undifferentiated unconscious,"* that is, as a mental level that unconsciously connects individuals.

And here the thought automatically goes to Bion's "protomental" (*"something in which the physical and the psychological or mental are in an undifferentiated state"*) and, along the Bionian lesson, to Jose Bleger's Symbiosis and Ambiguity, in which the Argentine psychoanalyst postulates the existence of a primitive "glischro-charged" position, which corresponds to a "symbiotic core" capable of immobilizing and controlling the psychotic part of the mind. A core that individuals "deposit" in institutions and, more generally, in the forms in which the life of a human society is organized. A deposit that collective catastrophes release with disastrous effects in society and the individuals who are part of it. In this regard, Silvia Amati Sas, a psychoanalyst, also from Argentina, but who has lived and worked in Italy for decades, has pointed to the attack on the Twin Towers as the cause of the collapse of the institutional repository that, in the era of globalization— not coincidentally, the towers housed the World Trade Center—had provided protection from the deep-seated anxieties generated by the mighty changes of our complex contemporaneity. The disappearance of this symbolic container is as if it had exposed us to that primitive, undifferentiated, magmatic and confusing emotional layer, from which we defend ourselves by building more mature processes, schizo-paranoid and depressive in nature, that make our relational and operational lives possible.

Also very interesting is the way in which the dreams received and "captured" in the matrices organized by the Authors at the height of the pandemic, when the world had all but stopped and frozen in a rigid lockdown, were analyzed as "texts" (as we are reminded about the semiotic approach) and re-signified in a sense-bearing narrative—K. Weick's sensemaking—and, in this way, to reconstruct the lived experience and to make possible transformative processes from which to start again in the time that remains to be lived.

The image of dream-catching, or rather dream-hunting, seems to me to have something to do with what Luigi Pagliarani taught us about the socioanalyzing element: a sign, a clue, most often a bizarre and distonic element within a narrative, but which, placed back into a new recomposed discourse, performs the function of a key able to make the whole comprehensible.

Also very beautiful is the image, drawn from the consideration that in ancient Egypt "one did not say 'having a dream,' as the dream was not an action, but instead 'seeing a dream,'" according to which the matrix represents, for those who participate in it and realize it, an experience analogous to that experienced by viewers of a film. In this regard, Cesare Musatti, psychoanalyst and cinephile, in describing the cinematic experience, reminded us of the interplay of cross-projections between the screen on which the images are projected and the spectators who in turn project their own fantasies stimulated by the images. To this exchange of projections, an additional element seems to be added with Social Dreaming, with the members of the group acting in turn as producers and projectionists of the images on the matrix screen.

I would like to conclude by returning to the authors' particularly timely reference to Ogden's lecture on the nature of thinking, between "magical," "oneiric," and "transformative thinking." The experience of Social Dreaming, properly structured and accompanied by a set of guiding theories and effective analytical tools, enables one to recursively traverse these three levels and forms of thinking, and to finally arrive at transformative thinking as a "*radically new way of organizing the experience.*" And to do so "*through dreams, nurtures creativity, imagination, individual responsibility, in a confrontation with the unconscious in which seeing one's own fears reflected in the eyes of the other allows a change of perspective and the build-ing of mutual bonds."*

A concrete possibility offered to those who propose to be able to succeed in pro-cessing together with other humans the collective traumas that reality replays to us repeatedly, but with unpredictable frequency, and that we can only hope to deal with to the extent that we will be able to think the unthinkable, being able to finally trans-form events into experience.

Psychosocioanalyst   Dario Forti
Founder of MODUS Benefit Society
Founder and Past President of Ariele (Italian
Association of Psychicosocioanalysis)
Milan, Italy
June 2023

Preface

This work begins in times of a pandemic to describe an experience of Social Dreaming that the two authors, Elisabetta Pasini and Cinzia Trimboli, hosted during the first lockdown in Italy, between early March and May 2020.

Suddenly, at that time, the COVID 19 emergency brought about a radical change in our lives, deeply affecting our inner psychological balance.

This work, however, grew out of an insight that prompted us to write at such a particular time: that the pandemic should not be seen merely as an upheaval of doom, but could have been instead an opportunity to develop a new and different way of thinking about ourselves and our actions in the world. We understand that this does not happen in solitude, but together with other people who have the same emotions, hopes, and fears, through complex interactions in a context that is constantly changing before our eyes.

The experience described in the following pages is the result of constant interactions aimed at combining our different backgrounds, skills, and experiences, as Jungian Psychoanalyst (Elisabetta) and as Psychologist and Researcher of narrative methodologies (Cinzia). In the development of the chapters we have chosen to cross-fertilize our expertise as much as possible, to make it easier for the reader to get the idea of a common project, the result of a professional collaboration that began a long time ago and has been strengthened over the past 2 years through the countless discussions and exchanges that enabled us to write these pages. This book starts therefore with the description of the experience of Social Dreaming we have done during the early days of the Covid-19 pandemic, when our lives had suddenly been completely subverted from one day to the other. It aims to tells the story of a journey of exploration we started in the darkest moments we've lived through at the beginning of the pandemic, that was a particularly difficult moment of bewilderment, in Italy and abroad. But this work also aims to combine two different and yet complementary perspectives on dream analysis, the analytical psychology of C.G. Jung and the narrative and semiotic approach of the social research, in the attempt to bring a contribution to the understanding of the changes that are taking place today in and around us. Chapter 1 therefore describes the methodology of Social Dreaming and its origins in the "milieu" of the social research at the beginning of the 19 century. Chapter 2 describes the elements of turbulence and the signs of change in the social context which were already found to be before the pandemic outbreak. Chapter 3 is the detailed, accurate description of the 4 Social Dreaming Matrices run between March and May 2020, including dreams, associations, amplifications and metaphors that were brought to light, and a final feedback from the participants. Chapter 5 describes the social function of dreams and the approach to dreams adopted by Jung's Analytical Psychology, bringing to light the figure of Gordon Lawrence, the founder of Social Dreaming. Chapter 6 describes the fundamentals of the narrative and the semiotic approach. Chapter 6 analyzes the EUNAMES case history, bringing to light how Social Dreaming can contribute to built a community of intents. Eventually, chapter 7 resumes the learnings and the discoveries made along the way, postulating a possible future for the Dream Journeys.

Finally, this work was made possible thanks to the contributions of the many fellow travelers who joined us on the journey. First of all, we would like to thank the group of adventurous "dream hunters" who gradually grew over the course of the four stages of the journey. The generosity with which each of them shared their dreams and the richness of their associations and amplifications are the most precious treasure of the journey. Special thanks go to Alessio Dammicco and Giulio Clemente, who were an integral part of the staff that worked on the dream narratives and made a valuable contribution in the film editing, supporting the oneiric scenes. Sincere thanks to those who have supported and encouraged us from a distance, in particular to Maria Giulia Marini of Eunames for the enthusiasm with which she involved us in a project that allowed us to consolidate our initial work; Micaela Castiglioni, Associate Professor at the University of Milano Bicocca, for her thoughtful inspirations; Dario Forti, who always supported our research as former President of Ariele, the Italian Association of Psychosocioanalysis; and Carlos Remotti Breton, President of OPUS, for the valuable work we have done together over the years on the development of Social Dreaming and Listening Post.

Milan, Italy   Elisabetta Pasini
Turin, Italy   Cinzia Trimboli

Contents

About the Authors

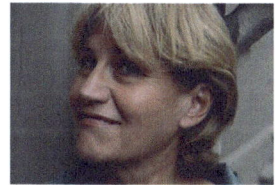 **Elisabetta Pasini** Jungian Psychoanalyst accredited at the Zurich C.G. Jung Institute for Analytical Psychology, Master in Social Anthropology at the London School of Economics, in my professional experience I have always been concerned with the development of individuals, groups, and organizations. In more than 15 years of living and working abroad (UK, US, Latin America, Switzerland, Spain, Dubai), I have gained significant experience in transcultural differences and their impact on the personal development of individuals.

Founder of The Flying Carpet Studio (www.theflyingcarpet.it), currently I live and work in Milan where I have my private practice as Psychoanalyst. Since 2018 I work at IMD Business School in Lausanne as Personal Development Analyst in the international MBA program, and with NAGA ONLUS in Milan to provide social, health, and psychological assistance to refugees and asylum seekers.

Memberships
- Member of IAAP—International Association for Analytical Psychology
- Member of OPUS—Organisation for Promoting Social Understanding in Society, London

Books and Articles
- Carisma, il Segreto del Leader—Garzanti, Milano, 2009
- Listening Post & Social Dreaming: esplorare l'immaginario sociale e stimolare la na-scita di un

nuovo pensiero collettivo—in Cantieri, Educazione
Sentimentale n. 33/2020—Franco Angeli, Milano

– Cinderella vs Sherazade: the Symbolic Meaning of
the Veil in the Islamic Culture—paper at the Opus
International   Conference,   London,   18/19
November 2016

– The Three Paradoxes of the Leaderless Organization,
in Organizational and Social Dynamics, vol. 15-1,
Karnac Books, London, 2015

– Charisma as Liminal Space: New Perspectives for
the Charismatic Phenomenon in the Digital Era,
paper at the Opus International Conference, London,
21/22 November 2014

– Conversations about Charisma: Andrea Branzi and
Bruce Mau, in Experimenta, July 2008

– Camper: from an Ethic of Process to an Ethic of
Concept, in Experimenta, October 2005

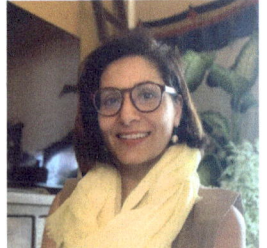

Cinzia Trimboli cinzia.trimboli@outlook.com – +39
3490641227

https://www.linkedin.com/in/cinzia-trimboli-
0b986a8/

Psychologist, my work experience began in corpo-
rate training in 2000 and then evolved into qualitative
research where I collaborate with market research insti-
tutes in the Italian and international scene.

Always passionate about social and organizational
research aimed at exploring emerging dynamics related
to change in 2014 I became a PSOA Counselor (following the psychosocioanalytic approach) for role counsel-
ing and organizational development and began
collaborating with Opus as part of Listening Post's
international research. In 2018, I began collaborating
with the Master in Training and Development of Human
Resources at the University of Milan Bicocca. Currently
a member of the Order of Psychologists of Piedmont
(OPO) and a member of OPUS (Organization for the
Promotion of the Understanding of Society). After the
experience of Social Dreaming during the lockdown,
The Flying Carpet project was born with Elisabetta
Pasini driven by the desire to continue to explore the
theme of moments of transition in the lives of individuals and the ways through which to support them.

My Background
- MA course in Applied Narrative Medicine, Istud, Milan Italia
- Training in Psychosocioanalysis—Ariele, Italian Association of Psychosocioanalysis, Milano, Italia
- MA course in Methodology of Applied Social and Market Research, Università Cattolica del Sacro Cuore, Milan, Italy
- Master's Degree in Labour and Organization Psychology, University of Turin, Italy

Books and Articles
- Edited by Dario Forti, Mauro Ceruti, Paolo Magatti, Daniela Patruno, Giorgio Puzzini, Paolo Romagnoli, Barbara Toffolo, Mauro Tomè, Cinzia Trimboli (2021) Cantieri. Un pedagogista geniale. Ricordando Paolo Perticari/Per il welfare che verrà. Agorà, uno spazio di ricerca e di intervento. In *Educazione Sentimentale*, 35, Franco Angeli, Milano
- Elisabetta Pasini, Cinzia Trimboli (2020) Listening Post & Social Dreaming: esplorare l'immaginario sociale e stimolare la nascita di un nuovo pensiero collettivo—in Cantieri, in *Educazione Sentimentale*, 33, Franco Angeli, Milano
- Baldassarre M., Trimboli C. (2014) Presenti sommersi, futuri emergenti: una lettura psicosocioanalitica dei cambiamenti individuali e collettivi, in *Educazione sentimentale*, 21, Franco Angeli, Milano
- Edited by Andrea Coco, Fabio Galluccio, Claudia Piccardo, Cinzia Trimboli (2009) Proposta di utilizzo del film "Un tocco di zenzero" a supporto della formazione al cambiamento, in *FOR Rivista per la formazione*, 80, Franco Angeli

Chapter 1
Introduction to Social Dreaming

The first chapter of this book is devoted to an overview of some of the most important elements that characterize the Social Dreaming methodology, which is at the center of our investigation, referring to the dedicated chapter for further discussion.

A brief history of the origins of Social Dreaming within the cultural milieu of the Tavistock Institute of Human Relations highlights how it has been used from the beginning in highly confrontational situations of collective trauma.

We refer here to the work of Riccardo Bernardini [1], who explores these aspects well, in a book dedicated to training methods [1].

Social Dreaming (SD) is a methodology that originated in 1982, thanks to W. Gordon Lawrence, in the cultural and professional context of the Tavistock Institute of Human Relations in London [2–4]. The origins of the Tavistock Institute date back to 1946, when a group of medical professionals of the Tavistock Clinic began working with the British Army to help soldiers who served in World War II to overcome the traumatic experience of the war and to return to a civilian life. The Tavistock Clinic's group included the most prestigious names in the field of psychiatry and psychoanalysis, such as Mary Ainsworth, Michael Balint, Wilfred Bion, John Bowlby, Martha Harris, Elliott Jaques, Donald Meltzer, and John Sutherland. The Tavistock Institute's renowned reputation stems from their work and is still active today as one of the most prominent institutions studying organizational change in work environments [5]. Social Dreaming plays a prominent role in its tradition.

The first Social Dreaming experiment was conducted in 1982 as part of the "Social Dreaming and Creativity Program" initiated by Gordon Lawrence with the official intent of conducting cultural inquiry through dreams [3]. The sequence of the sessions was named the Social Dreaming Matrices (SDM), and Lawrence adopted the term matrix to refer to the network of existing minds that, at any given time, are driven to focus on a particular topic.

© The Author(s), under exclusive license to Springer Nature
Switzerland AG 2023
E. Pasini, C. Trimboli, *A Social Dreaming Experience at the Time of COVID 19*,
New Paradigms in Healthcare, https://doi.org/10.1007/978-3-031-42498-4_1

Gordon Lawrence took the world "matrix" from the work of Siegfried Heinrich Foulkes, who firstly introduced the concept of "matrix" in the psychodynamic field of studies [6]. Foulkes was a group psychoanalyst and called matrix an intangible element that characterizes group situations, that is, a kind of shared common ground that shapes the meaning and signification of events and on which all verbal and non-verbal communication rests, in which individuals are notational points of the network of the matrix.

Lawrence's idea of the mind of the group was also strongly influenced by Kurt Lewin pioneer work in Social Psychology. Lewin was the first to theorize the existence of a group thinking with its own characteristics, capable of autonomous psychic manifestations [7].

Finally, we may recall that the etymology of the word "matrix" comes from the Latin word "uterus," "mother," "origin," to mean, as suggested by Gordon Lawrence contributor Patricia Daniel, "a generative place from which something is born" [8, p. 39].

The "Social Dreaming and Creativity Program" initiated by Lawrence ran for 8 weeks, with weekly meetings of one and a half hours, and was attended by 13 people with different professional backgrounds. In each Social Dreaming session chairs were arranged in spiral, so that people were placed at different angles and had their backs to each other, with no direct eye contact. In the meetings, participants were asked to share dreams, provide associations to the dreams of others, to explore the outcomes of possible social meaning. At the end of the experiment, Lawrence and Daniel concluded, "It can be hypothesized with greater consistency that it is possible to have dreams that speak to our unconscious fears and anxieties about the society in which we live" [2, p. 80].

In Lawrence's idea, Social Dreaming was therefore a useful tool to explore the social meanings of the dreams made available in the matrix, bringing dreams out of the "analysis room" and restoring the social function they had in the past to facilitate the formation of shared collective thinking and the creation of social bonds and connections [3, 9]. After the first successful experience conducted by Lawrence, Social Dreaming was widely used in training, organizational consulting projects, high conflicting situations, international scenarios forecasting, highlighting many points of contact with C.G. Jung's Analytical Psychology approach.

Today, Social Dreaming is widely used in organizational projects to delve on topics of leadership and innovation. Since 1988, several Social Dreaming programs have been developed in various countries around the world (Israel, Germany, Sweden, UK, Belgium, India, Australia, and the USA), arousing interest and recognition at an international level [3, 10]. Its applications are found in a wide variety of contexts: educational, welfare, vocational, community [11–13].

The four main cornerstones of Social Dreaming can be defined as follows [1].

First, the dreams shared in the matrix contain information about the collective psychic dimension (group, organizational, or social) in which the dreamers are embedded.

Living beings interact within a context and are expression of that same context.

When we dream, therefore, we are in relation not only to our inner world, but also to the external world [14]. C.G. Jung speaks of a collective unconscious, to which, in his view, "big dreams" testify. The collective unconscious speaks through archetypal images that inhabit the deepest structure of psychic life and tend to surface especially at decisive moments in life, conveying a message that has collective value. Big dreams contain therefore "a collective meaning," which is at the same time an expression of value not only for the subject itself, but also of the fact that "the problem of the individual, at that moment, is also a problem of the collective" [15, pp. 220].

Second, the matrix collects "emergent" contents, not yet surfaced to consciousness.

According to Lawrence's thinking in the dream we find an anticipatory valence of our being in the world [8]. Claudio Neri, psychoanalyst and group psychotherapist, says that "it is as if people who dream [...] are able to grasp evidence that those who are awake cannot or do not want to see. The eyes of the dreamer are probably removed from the constraints of the social group and can therefore see facts, forces and tensions that the eyes of those who are awake cannot recognize" [5, p. 49].

Third, the matrix evokes a different kind of dreams than other "containers," such as dual analysis or group psychotherapy.

In the current psychoanalytical practice dreams analysis occurs mainly in a dual setting centered on the interpretation of the latent significance of the dream, in order to overcome patient's trauma. Lawrence's dream work is different, as dreams in the matrix allow participants to learn from others through free associations, amplifications, and systemic thinking, encouraging spontaneity and the expression of creative responses to dream imagery. Interpretation in the classical psychoanalytic sense is not allowed either with regard to dream content or group dynamics. In Social Dreaming, in fact, the dreams that are shared in the matrix are communal, not a "private property" of the dreamer [5, p. 52].

Fourth, the work in the matrix focuses on the dream rather than the dreamer.

The experience of the Social Dreaming Matrix aims to increase awareness through developmental thinking that is not anchored to consciousness and rational thinking, but is rather capable to evolve facing uncertainty and paradox. The metaphor of the matrix as a "womb" is in this sense particularly evocative as a generative fertile space.

In summary, the development of Social Dreaming was, in Gordon Lawrence's belief, a way to gain an in-depth understanding of the life of organizations through the dream lives of the people in them, in order to reveal the blind side that lurks in every organization [14], beyond what is visible, logical, and rational. When, at certain times in the life of an organization, tensions and conflicts are pushed to the highest levels, the Western myth of rational control proves to be a pure illusion and it becomes necessary to adopt a questioning approach. Which is, as Neri suggests, letting the unexpressed questions of the organization come to the surface, which can be more useful and effective than looking for ready-made answers; a useful "antidote to the sterility of organizations' dialogues [...] in times of conservative stagnation and asphyxiation of thought" [16, p. 23].

Social Dreaming represents an appropriate space to accommodate such "questions," allowing people to relate to them and try to process them. The exploration of dreams represents the right "container" for the creative potential of the collective unconscious: an exploration of what is unspoken, and presumably unknown, but could reveal fears, fantasies, and internal conflicts, leading at the same time to a better understanding of the organizational reality [17].

As anticipated, there are several areas of application.

Dreams have always been a valuable path of knowledge, and over time dreaming has been used by many cultures around the world as an important way to capture thinking about the past and learning about the present, guiding people into the future. Social Dreaming builds on this legacy to bring new thinking and meaning to the contemporary society in which we live and work.

Social Dreaming is used in organizations, groups, associations, communities, projects, events, conferences, or stand-alone forums for discovering the communal meaning in our dreams. Opening our minds to dreams by sharing them with others generates new thinking, makes us discover new sources of knowledge, opens the mind to different perspectives.

Social Dreaming is an enjoyable and revealing experience in which participants learn to think divergently, breaking with the more typical discourse of goal orientation.

The associative process of the matrix allows open, nonjudgmental expression of thoughts, enabling participants to promote free thinking and social interaction to co-create new meanings.

Aware of the richness of this methodology, at the dawn of 2020, we had planned to organize a Social Dreaming Matrix as part of a research project on psychosocial trends through the investigation of the social meaning of dreams.

The rapid and unexpected spread of the COVID-19 pandemic and the exceptional nature of the lockdown that brought Italy to a halt in early 2020 abruptly changed our plans. All in-person activities had been banned. At the same time, however, we thought that the pandemic could have been an opportunity to test in a new and highly traumatic context a methodology we had been working on for some time. At a time of great confusion and bewilderment, looking at dreams as catalysts for change, and dreamtime as a space of transition, had seemed to us the only possible way to make sense of what was happening around us.

Three years have passed since then.

In May 2023, the World Health Organization's announcement marked the official end of the state of emergency due to the pandemic, which almost sounds like a release.

It took 1221 days, as many as have passed since that January 30, 2020, the official date of entry into the COVID nightmare. History tells us of nearly 800 million confirmed COVID-19 cases worldwide since the pandemic began and officially nearly 7 million deaths. In Italy we had almost 26 million cases and close to 190,000 victims.

In the words of Tedros Ghebreyesus, director of WHO, making the long-awaited announcement, however, there is a cautious optimism: "It is with great hope that I now declare the end of Covid-19 as a global health emergency, but that does not mean that Covid is over in terms of its threat to global health."

The publication of this paper is an opportunity to bring the collective experience of the pandemic back to memory, bringing into focus some of the questions that the dream imagery of the time brought to light. Hoping that this contribution will help to reflect on the possibilities of following up on change, and the need to transform our thinking about the world in a rapidly changing context.

References

1. Bernardini R. Social dreaming. In: Quaglino GP, editor. Formazione. I metodi. Milano: Raffaello Cortina Editori; 2020. p. 789–813.
2. Lawrence WG. Ventures in social dreaming. Changes. 1989;7(3):3–25.
3. Lawrence WG. Won from the void and formless infinite: experiences of social dreaming. Free Assoc. 1991;2(2):259–94.
4. Lawrence WG, Daniel P. A venture in social dreaming. London: Tavistock Documents; 1982.
5. Neri C. Presentazioni del metodo e della tecnica del Social dreaming. 2003.
6. Foulkes SH. Analisi terapeutica di gruppo. Tr. it. Torino: Bollati Boringhieri; 1964. p. 1967.
7. Lewin K, Cartwright D. Field theory in social science. New York: Harper; 1951.
8. Lawrence WG. Social dreaming. La funzione sociale del sogno. Roma: Borla; 2001.
9. Lawrence WG. The social dreaming matrix for the transformation of thinking and the awakening of shadows. FOR. 2006;67:64–71.
10. Lawrence WG. Social dreaming as a tool of consultancy and action research. In: Sievers B, et al., editors. Psychoanalytic studies of organizations. Contributions from the International Society for the Psychoanalytic Study of Organizations (ISPSO). London: Karnac; 2009. p. 105–22.
11. Lawrence WG, editor. Esperienze nel social dreaming. Tr. it. Roma: Borla; 2003a. p. 2004.
12. Lawrence WG, editor. Infinite possibilities of social dreaming. Londra: Karnac; 2007.
13. Lawrence WG, editor. The creativity of social dreaming. London: Karnac; 2010.
14. Lawrence WG. Social dreaming as sustained thinking. Hum Relat. 2003b;56(5):609–24.
15. Jung CG. Il significato della psicologia per i tempi moderni. Tr. it. In: Opere, vol. 10. Torino: Bollati Boringhieri; 1933–1934. p. 1985.
16. Garofalo N. Social dreaming, un fraintendimento virtuoso nel nome. FOR. 2012;92:23–6.
17. Gasseau M, Bernardini R. Il sogno. Dalla psicologia analitica allo psicodramma junghiano. Milano: Franco Angeli; 2009.

Chapter 2
Dreams and Collective Trauma

2.1   An Adventurous Journey

> There is a story to tell. It tells about the sea, a group of men and a quest. There is a boat, Argo, with valiant and courageous heroes aboard; some say that there were forty eight, others say fifty five. What's for certain is that their names were never forgotten. Hercules, Castor, Atalanta, Laertes, Orpheus, Erialus, Euphemus etc. Their leader was Jason, the son of Aeson, descendant of Aeolus, the god of wind. They set forth with one objective: to seize the Golden Fleece, the coat of a flying ram symbol of power that would enable Jason to reclaim his kingdom that was unfairly usurped by his uncle Pelia. The precious trophy was kept in a faraway land, and in order to reach it, one had to cross a sea full of perils and difficulties. Everyone thought that this voyage was impossible, foolhardy, too dangerous.
>
> AA.VV. [1] Argo. A modern story, beyond sailing

One of the most fascinating myths of antiquity, the expedition of the Argonauts in search of the Golden Fleece celebrates the deeds of the most extraordinary talents of the ancient Greece, like Heracles the invincible hero, Orpheus the cantor of the gods, the Dioscuri twins Castor and Pollux, and many others.

What did the 50 heroes have to prove when they sailed with the ship Argo to the Colchis, a faraway country on the edge of the world, following Jason, a reckless young man without a kingdom, whose only merit was owning a beautiful boat and having a destiny? All of them were already famous; many of them left a kingdom, a family, lot of certainties; some of them did not return. However, all of them were driven by the same urgency to start the journey, accomplishing the deed, challenging fate.

Generally, it is in situations of change that the impulse to challenge habitual patterns of thinking, changing the usual life strategies, seeking creative solutions in the new scenarios of personal and working life, is most keenly felt.

The difficult period we experienced during the pandemic was one such moment, when the fears and anxieties unleashed began to question our future and the fragile balance on which global society rests.

E. Pasini, C. Trimboli, *A Social Dreaming Experience at the Time of COVID 19*,
New Paradigms in Healthcare, https://doi.org/10.1007/978-3-031-42498-4_2

The arrival of the pandemic in Italy in January 2020 found us unprepared, disbelieving and helpless in the face of the scope and speed of the spread of the contagion, and, especially in the regions of northern Italy most adversely affected by the pandemic, it was a traumatic element in terms of the impact on people's lives.

The ISTAT[1] report of May 3, 2021 contains some data collected by the Integrated National Surveillance System of the Italian National Institute of Health: in 2020 there was an increase of +112,000 deaths over the previous year, of which 75,891 were directly attributable to COVID-19 and recorded by health authorities. The paper also speculates that an additional portion of deaths were caused by other lethal diseases, which could not be adequately treated by our National Health System struggling with the ongoing emergency.

Against this chaotic backdrop in the initial phase, an optimistic expectation seemed to make its way to a part of civil society, represented by the slogans hung on balconies, "Everything will be fine," which wished the return to a new normality and the recovery of the lifestyle to which we were accustomed.

At the same time, the situation opened up great questions about the future to come. The "bubble" in which we were imprisoned waiting for the wave to pass fueled the desire to break out of the stalemate, activating resources to react to the flow of events and alarming news coming from outside. Some argued that nothing would ever be the same again. Many felt the urge to imagine new life scenarios, stimulated by the challenge of exploring new unknown territories.

The pandemic thus became an opportunity for a journey of discovery, a challenge from which to expect new knowledge, according to Frank's [2] scheme applied to story analyses. An elective way to initiate a search for meaning and awareness, through a reflection that would put people's subjective experiences at the center.

The idea of starting a Social Dreaming Matrix project in the initial phase of that period responded to this desire for questioning and personal activation, together with the possibility of not being alone in facing the unexpected. Like modern-day Argonauts, we embarked on a journey with an uncertain destination, moved by the desire and urgency to do something, as well as the need to share our experience with others. The decision to run four Social Dreaming Matrices online during the first stages of the pandemic was therefore the result of an intuition rather than a plan: exploring the dreams during the time of the 2020 first lockdown in Italy was our way to search for meanings face to unexpected overwhelming events, as well as an attempt to reconstruct the lost connections between the inner and the outer world.

The participants and travel companions who gradually joined us were mostly professionals who from one day to the next had been forced to think in isolation on how to reinvent their work.

---

[1]The National Institute of Statistics (ISTAT) is an Italian public research organization that conducts general censuses of population, services and industry, agriculture, household sample surveys, and general economic surveys at the national level. The data cited refer to the report published online on the institutional website: https://www.istat.it/it/files//2021/05/REPORT_INDICATORI-DEMOGRAFICI-2020.pdf

Right from the start, the journey meant relying on dreams and imagination, in the absence of established points of reference. This is how it all began. When asked therefore what we had seen in the dreams, we answered that it had been like embarking on an adventurous journey, a kind of parallel path in which "the order of the night" was a safe container that acted as a counterpoint, like a parallel world, to the increasingly problematic "order of the day."

We came across a surprising material both for the richness and evocative scope of the images and for the choral and dynamic nature of the narrative. Individual dreams naturally seemed to develop into a more collective and shared narrative.

Systematizing what we had done went hand in hand with the awareness that we were dealing with an extraordinary body of material, not so much (or not only) because of our own merit, but because of the extraordinary historical moment we were living.

The difficulty of reconnecting today, almost 3 years later, with those contents and experiences speaks volumes about the distance that has been created in memory and the desire for removal and return to normality. Many consider it a period of "freezing" of one's life. Yet it was precisely during that period, so distressingly charged with uncertainty and death, that new creative energies were unleashed, along with an awareness of our limits as human beings and of being part of a common destiny.

I still remember with goosebumps the first dream matrix of March 17. We were in full health emergency in Italy and the world. A domestic imagery "contaminated" by wild elements and negative omens emerged powerfully, straining the sense of individual and family security: large birds with huge beaks, fallen teeth, dried figs on the table, etc. The sense of death and threat was very present. The capacity for action in the social sphere seemed blocked, frozen: the landscape appeared motionless and empty, like the fruit of a spell. We found ourselves deprived of some certainties that had been solid up to that moment: tasting glasses shattered, fast cars lost pieces in their rush. The gaze seemed to turn mostly inward. Images of secret gardens appeared, crystal-clear waters to draw from, places reminiscent of a forgotten world where rebirth is possible, as well as finding the energy to re-imagine ourselves. This world, however, was not yet accessible.

Two weeks later, on April 1, the Matrix presented the clash between Nature and Culture. The symbols and signs of an ancient and archaic civilization were threatened by a looming nature silently occupying our spaces. The outdoor landscape became surreal; we saw men swimming in the subway, ivy-shrouded bookcases, men standing still in pools of water hiding in the forest. There were openings with cakes made of paper, lectures with no speaker to speak. There was a widespread sense of inadequacy. A recurring dream was about the difficulty of finding the right clothes to attend meetings; we were clumsy and awkward in our actions. We no longer knew what we could or could not do. We have sought refuge in small comfort objects, such as a shell necklace. However, we felt inside a dimension of stalemate, of imprisonment, from which it was difficult to find the way that, discarding things aside, would lead us to salvation.

The third Matrix, dated April 15, marks the end of the standoff. We were close to the end of the stalemate and the newspapers were already talking about reopening and restarting. In dreams, the contrast emerged between the threatening and complex reality before us and the longing for an ideal world to return to, far away and hard to reach. In the dreams, we were setting out again into a world that seemed warped, oppressive, claustrophobic. It was not clear where to go, nor what known means we could rely on. Unknown travelers showed us the way through a forest, a subway line. We left our luggage on the ground and climbed the most disparate and unlikely means. The landscape we traversed was grotesque, with soldiers transforming into clowns, elderly women struggling with giant light bulbs, giant buildings looming ominously, crowded with people celebrating at windows and oblivious to the danger of falling. The streets were deserted. The dungeons were filled with set tables to be carefully avoided. The journey undertaken appeared strenuous, expensive, uncertain, confronting us with unknown aspects. To sustain us and give us hope, a few colorful T-shirts, the song of whales," and the memory of the sea, an image repeatedly evoked and a symbol of a utopian world to strive toward.

Thus we arrived on May 5, at the dawn of phase 2, our last Matrix. Dreams spoke to us of a new sensory experience with the flavor of newfound freedom. Colors became vivid, we immersed ourselves in warm, jelly-like waters, the experience was almost hallucinatory. We stroked soft, zippered sheep coats, and flew through the air flapping our arms. The journey became a search for meanings. In dreams we would sort through books, give explanations, get back on the road. Beautiful young pregnant women embodied the strong expectations of rebirth. However, we were hesitant in the face of the bridges breaking in the void. We waited for a film director who never came, and in the air hovered a sense of unease, of threat, of abuse on our most fragile part. We could only count on one eye, the other was stitched shut. The dreams guided us to ask a question that became critical in those days: how capable are we of seeing what is in front of us? Furthermore, is our interaction with reality driven by the ability to rethink and reinvent the future or is it influenced by what we already know and can control?

The Social Dreaming experience that is the object of this book aims to show the importance imagination has on our capacity to deal with a highly traumatic collective situation such as the one experienced during the pandemic.

2.2   The Social Context of the COVID-19 Pandemic: The International Listening Post Project

Even before the Pandemic, an unusual seismic activity could be recorded where a certain asymptomatic collective feeling overflowed to generate History. Within a short time, several mythical figures of remarkable proportions began to reshape, as if propelled by a sudden urgency, the mental skyline of humans. While the digital revolution was unstoppably building across the planet the myth par excellence, that of a promised land, in more circumscribed areas of the world, great mythological tales of splendid craftsmanship were flourishing: the war on terror, then the threat of migrants, then the emergence of climate change, with a great classic in prospect: the end of the world. After decades of apparent

mythic anemia, some subterranean magma of very high temperature seemed to have found the mouth from which to erupt - roars and glows. Then, the Pandemic.
   Alessandro Baricco [3], Quel che Stavamo aspettando (What we were waiting for).

At the beginning of 2020 the pandemic took us by surprise.

When, in late 2019 and early 2020, the coronavirus started to infect and kill thousands of people from a Chinese market in the populous city of Wuhan, we could not at first believe that the virus would spread so rapidly among the whole world's population, country by country, at a much faster rate than we could have imagined.

We could not even imagine, at first, that the severe restrictive measures taken by the governments of the various countries that were progressively affected by the pandemic would have such a profound impact on our way of life.

The restrictive measures adopted by the governments were certainly justified by the exponential growth of the contagion, and in some cases as Italy, the first European country to be profoundly affected by a high number of deaths, had a profound impact on the daily living and working habits and, in the long term, on the mental health of certain sections of the population.

Just to give few examples of the measures that were taken at that time in Italy, we may remember that all kinds of social activities were abruptly suspended from 1 day to another, and people, with few exceptions, were forced to stay at home indefinitely; schools and universities were closed, children and adolescents obliged to online learning; the majority of the offices and production activities adopted extensive smart working measures from home; all kinds of outdoor leisure activities were suspended; shops were closed; trains, planes, public transports cancelled until further notice, and traveling from one city to another within the country was strictly forbidden. Among the different age groups, the youngest and the elderlies suffered the most for the forced isolation, many of the latter dying alone in retirement homes, away from family members and deprived of the rituals of funeral and burials, a vacuum that has not yet been filled. We all are still dealing with the dramatic images, impressed in our eyes, of exhausted health staff in hospitals covered from top to toe with medical garments and masks to protect themselves from the virus; and with the impressive number of stacked coffins transported by military tracks, waiting to be buried in large new cemeteries.

This abrupt dramatic suspension of the normal rhythm of life, both at a personal and collective level, for an indefinite period of time, was called "the lockdown."

The COVID-19 pandemic had a severe impact on the mental health and well-being of people around the world. A study of the World Health Organization (WHO), published on March 2022, underlines the early evidence of the impact of the pandemic on mental health.[2] COVID 19, outlines the study, led to an increase worldwide in 2020 of major depressive disorder (+27.6% on average), anxiety disorders (+25.6% on average), and an additional substantial Disability-Adjusted Life Years (DALYs) per 100,000 population. The greatest increases were found in places

---

[2] Mental Health and COVID-19: Early Evidence of the Pandemic's Impact, World Health Organization, 2 March 2022.

highly affected by COVID-19, females were more affected than males, and younger people, especially those aged 20–24 years, were more affected than older adults; low- and middle-income countries were also majorly affected. Major key-findings also underline a higher risk of an impact of the pandemic on suicidal behaviors among young people, and an increased risk for suicidal thoughts due to exhaustion (in healthcare workers), loneliness and positive COVID-19 diagnosis. Evidence suggests the pandemic led to a worldwide increase in mental health problems, including widespread depression and anxiety. People living with pre-existing mental disorders are also at greater risk of severe illness and death from COVID-19 and should be considered a risk group upon diagnosis of infection. Overall, data indicated that suicide rates in most countries did not rise early in the pandemic. However, the increased risk in young people and the longer-term impact of the pandemic on economic recession remains a concern on mental health and suicide rates, given the well-recognized link between suicidal behaviors and economic hardship. Overall, one could say that the pandemic has pervasively affected the "social bonds" that unite people, suddenly and unexpectedly highlighting the profound inequalities and limitations of our living and relationship system in terms of economic, social, gender and age gaps [4].

Going back to the end of 2019 and the beginning of 2020 I remember great concerns about the many signs of crisis spreading in the social context. Their strength and evidence make it difficult now, with hindsight, to argue that what happened in the aftermath of the pandemic was entirely unpredictable and totally unexpected. In the following we report a brief summary of the results of a global social research program, the International Listening Post project,[3] to which I have been working since 2012 as member of OPUS, to highlight the huge impact that the anxieties and concerns already present in the social context at the beginning of 2020 had on people's everyday lives.

Listening Post (LP) and Social Dreaming (SD) were born in the late 1970s and early 1980s from the same cultural environment, the Tavistock Institute for Human Relations in London.

Building on the experiences and research conducted by the British psychoanalyst Wilfred Bion on individuals and groups at the beginning of the 19 century, the Tavistock Institute launched in the 70s the famous Leicester Conferences, wherein its tradition of group relations in organizational and institutional contexts was applied to the development of specific methodologies, aimed to increase the self-awareness and the reflective capacities of individuals and groups.

The two devices, Listening Post and Social Dreaming, have, therefore, a common origin, but also some major differences, that refer to what we might call the "order of the day" (LP), focused on the experience of the individuals as citizens living and acting in a social context; and the "order of the night," the shared

---

[3] OPUS, Organisation for Promoting the Social Understanding of Society, since 1975 promotes studies and researches to understand the dynamics of change in the society. OPUS runs every year the International Listening Post, regular meetings that take a 'snapshot' of society at a particular moment in time, taking place at the same time in more than 30 countries in the world.

narrative of the dreaming experience of the individuals in a group (SD). Those two levels of experience are different but complementary, and the combined use of both allows to deal with social phenomena from an inner and an outer perspective, and to connect the whole experience of the subject.

We will explore in details the many aspects of the Social Dreaming, which is the main focus of this work, in the next chapters of this book. Let us focus our attention now on the Listening Post methodology, developed by OPUS—*Organization for Promoting the Social Understanding of Society*, a non-profit organization established in the early 1980s as a spin-off of the Tavistock Institute, with the specific function of observing and interpreting the signs of change in the broader social context.

The basic idea that stands behind the LP derives from the theory of complex systems, according to which a group of people that come together to analyze the behavior of a society as such allows for the unconscious expression of certain characteristics of the extended social system (isomorphism).

The first Listening Post related experiments have been developed at the Tavistock in the early 1980s by Eric Miller and Olya Khaleelee, building on Bion's legacy on the observation of the social context, beginning with an aspect that Bion himself had at the time only hinted at. The extended social context, says Bion, can be observed as an intelligible system by adopting a "satellite" view on reality [5]. That is, reality is composed by a constellation of interconnected points of view that observe the social context itself and the processes of change taking place in a given temporal frame. The project was carried out as an attempt to implement a method of observation and intervention in the society, that could facilitate the expression and the interpretation of conscious and unconscious processes in complex organizational systems.

OPUS was established, therefore, in these years as an observatory on social change to explore the social dynamics in a group representative of an extended system. The internal cohesion and motivation of the participants was found in their common characteristic of "reflective citizens," active members of a community, who have a critical view on the social issues at stake and are looking for new ways to impact and involvement.

The observation of the social context as a whole is based on the Bion's theory of the development of thoughts as a recursive thinking/linking process [6]. New thoughts are developed through the connections and associations made in a group that enable people to cope with feelings of frustrations, absence, lack of meaning, activating the capacity of symbolization.

Since 2012 I have been working both with OPUS and *Ariele, the Italian Association of Psychosocio analysis*, in applying Listening Post to different organizational contexts, in order to observe and better understand the signals of change in society.

Since 2012 in fact Ariele has taken part in the OPUS' International Observatory on Social Change, regular meetings that are held in around 30 countries in the world in January of each year under the guidance and coordination of OPUS, to take a "snapshot" of the society at a particular moment of time. The constant monitoring of the issues at stake at the time in the different social contexts and the comparison of the results allow to have a historical survey on the psychosocial trends of change [7, 8].

We are living in years of rapid and sudden change, exposed to life experiences that mark the transition from what we thought was a stable and secure way of life, to a world which is charged of deep unknown. Uncertainties and insecurity about the future solicit strong anxieties and fears, but they may also give rise to hopes and projects, in only we were able to deal with them. Face to the challenges of our time, I believe that the development of an individual reflective capacity is essential for a better understanding of both the rational and the emotional issues, starting from the belief that, to build a better future for all of us, "head and the heart" should walk together.

Back to the OPUS' International Observatory on Social Change, we have already pointed out that a regular monitoring of the emerging signals of change has been made, since 2003, running yearly sessions of Listening Post in more than 30 countries in the world.

Let us have a closer look now to the details of the LP methodology, which we have so far discussed only in its general characters.

The underlying assumption of the LP is that in social systems in transition change occurs simultaneously at two different levels:

- **the social level**, which includes products, services, technology, social organization, culture, roles, procedures, etc.;
- **the psychological level**, which includes beliefs, values, hopes, anxieties, defense mechanisms, and ways of thinking of the individuals, which determine how they perceive the external reality and shape their actions.

These two levels are constantly interacting, and what goes on in people's minds is both reactive to what is going on around them and proactive in the sense that it can influence and direct the changes that are taking place. We have already pointed out that LP starts from the assumption that a group of people that come together to analyze the behavior of a society as such, enables the unconscious expression of certain characteristics of the extended social system.

The main objective of the LP is thus to enable participants, as individuals and "reflective citizens," to exchange their experience and concerns within the social context, in an enough safe and secure setting that allows free expression and encourages to take taking a perspective of "active agents of change."

In a LP session participants have the opportunity to test their abilities to:

- grasp and elaborate the so-called weak signals of change
- broaden their point of view, through the discussion in a heterogeneous group
- reflect on the emerging causes that provoke change and the hidden defenses that may hinder it

Each LP session is composed of 12–15 participants, heterogeneous in terms of age, gender, personal and professional experience, to provide a sufficiently representative cross-section of society.

Each LP session lasts 2.5 h, is coordinated by a "convener," and is divided into three phases, each of one of them with different objectives:

- in phase 1 participants share their experiences and concerns in a free session of "brainstorming" (1 h)
- in phase 2 participants, divided in small groups, highlight the main themes emerged from the discussion in phase 1 (30′)
- in phase 3, in plenary, they make hypothesis on what is going on at a conscious and unconscious level in society (1 h)

To better orient the reader, we provide below some brief examples of the connections between the micro- and macro-phenomena of change that have been detected at different levels over the past few years.

In the area of the Subject we observed that the "fear of the foreigners," linked with the exponential growth of migrations in the more recent years, has been emphasized as a great concern that have serious impact in the daily life of people since 2013. Its roots can be traced in a systemic crisis, experienced by the individuals as lack of opportunities, heightened over time by uncertain life conditions, cause of a profound mistrust in institutions and politics, leading to lose hope toward the future. The external reality is experienced as threatening, persecutory, social relations limited to distant connections in a virtual universe. Isolated individuals try to protect themselves living in the reassuring "bubble," of their daily life, withdrawing from social engagement and responsibility.

In the Social area, the long-lasting lack of dialogue between generations causes an age conflict that is more evident over the years, ending into a "gerontocracy" with has a strong defensive character, where the elders hold privileges they are unwilling to lose, to the detriment of the younger generations. As a result, any social instance of renewal is stuck, any political decision proves ineffective and fails to translate into concrete actions and new perspectives. The past is seen as a mythological happy Eden, and the desire to belong to a community covers the need to take refuge against creeping loneliness and anomy.

Technology and the media, since 2012, have been blamed as the main cause of issues like the distortion of communication, the verbal aggressiveness, anger and frustration. Widespread feelings of "living in combat," bring people to adhere to false models. The hyper-technological reality heightens people's constant swinging between delusions of omnipotence and feelings of powerlessness, between the need to be always connected and the wish to be able to disconnect from everything and everyone.

Finally, the most problematic area of life concerns social and political engagement. People question if a European Community with a common history really exists. At a deepest level change is identified with the end of an era, represented by the image of a complex Babel of languages, deprived of common values. Migrants seem to be the sole carriers of some kind of authenticity. Puzzling parallels, such as that between "autism and activism" embodied by the figure of the child Greta

Thunberg, hark back to the specter of a political power sick with infantilism, incapable of handling an environmental catastrophe.

This was the world "before COVID 19" as it looked at the dawn of 2020, when the pre-pandemic LP session was held in Milan. Images of a jumble of fears and hopes, in which some suggestions, however, prove to be, with the eyes of the aftermath, truly illuminating.

As final stage of the analysis, let us therefore have a glimpse of the main themes that emerged in the Listening Post session of January 2020, just before the pandemic outbreak.

2.2.1   Flanerie, or the Search for Meaning in a Changing World

The image of the "flaneur," the lonely wanderer in the urban drift, with no intention or desire, is the protagonist of the poetic attitude made famous in the early 1900s by the French poet Baudelaire. "Flanerie" underlines a covered need for emotion and surprise, represents a metaphor for an exploratory attitude aimed at achieving a new sense of reality, looking at it with new eyes. A new existentialism that wants to make room for a reflective attitude, recovering individual capacity for action in the sphere in which one lives and works, together with others who share the same values. Reality may be problematic, harsh, threatening. But the antidote to isolation and loneliness is an inclusive community of intent, open to the acceptance of differences.

2.2.2   We Need an Exoskeleton

Face to the increasing complexity of the technological world, the balance between new options and frightening issues is complex. Fake news make impossible to distinguish between true and false, scientific expertise is underestimated. But a purely defensive attitude does not help. What we need instead is an "exoskeleton" like that of the shrimps, an armor to protect ourselves that could also help us to walk. If we have lost control upon reality, we may accept the idea that we lack of something, that we need a container for the strong emotions—anxieties, aggression, fears—making us less permeable to external harm. A container capable of uniting the dots of individual solitudes, of making us feel no longer like isolated "bits" scattered in a virtual universe, but like "lego cubes" that fit together to give each other mutual support.

2.2.3   The Interregnum and the Shapeshifter

We are living an interregnum, in an in-between world in constant transition. But this world is crowded with figures, images, heroic characters. Most importantly, we can be in it, we are those lego cubes, those little dots, those sardines who have learned to swim and are now looking for direction in an unstable universe—in Italy the so-called sardine movement was at that time at its peak, a spontaneous movement that brought large numbers of people into the squares, eager to lay the foundations of a new sociality. We can find direction and meaning in continuous change, the coexistence of opposites is possible, if only we can free ourselves from the logic of polarization, the logic of war, and rediscover relationships of mutual trust.

This was the "spirit of the time" at the outbreak of the pandemic, which erupted like a collective trauma. The main most visible effect of a traumatic experience is the block of the capacity to act. Face to a traumatic situation everything goes to a halt, the passing of time freezes in an endless repetition of the same single moment, future and past coexist in an eternal present, the traumatic experience is endlessly repeated. The experience of trauma cuts the link with the world as a defense against an overly threatening reality. We feel trapped in a dead-end situation that annihilates our ability to think and relate, the faculties of symbolization and imagination blocked by fear.

However, hope arises that fears could heighten the collective awareness of our singular vulnerability, giving a boost to the urgency of recovering bonds of solidarity and common values. Like the Naomi Klein describes in her book *The Shock Doctrine*, in which the violence produced by the catastrophes and totalitarianisms of the last century—from the putsch in Chile to the tsunami in Thailand—instead of destroying existing social bonds, gave rise to "solidarity antibodies" among people. Or the biblical fear as engine of knowledge described by the American political scientist Corey Robin, which has its roots in Adam and Eve's expulsion from the Garden of Eden, whose echo resonates in the Bible's fateful phrase: "Through fear they know."

Fear releases energy, we must learn to use it, headlined a popular Italian newspaper in June 2021.

Our hyper-connected digital world provides many contents, but few containers for the co-creation of common experiences.

In the following pages we will try to highlight how Social Dreaming could be such a safe container for the development of new forms of intimacy and sociability, enabling people to overcome a traumatic situation through the sharing of dreams.

2.3 The Loss of Habits, the Discovery of Habitat

> To see a landscape we must have already dreamed it: the landscape is not only that portion
> of nature that shows itself to us today. It is the invisible place where the external world and
> the psychic world meet and merge, ushering in new boundaries.
>   Vittorio Lingiardi [9], Mindscapes

When we found ourselves locked in our homes, I remember that one of the strongest
experiences I had, beyond the fear of contagion and serious consequences for me
and my family, having elderly parents, was a sense of estrangement from the dimensions of time and space I had been familiar with up to that point.

Suddenly we found ourselves deprived of our habits, our rhythms, the small and
large rituals of the daily routine. The first phase of the lockdown was disorienting in
that it freed up time and at the same time forced action into the domestic context.

The forced stop for COVID was experienced by many as an event that interrupted a daily routine, dreams and plans, posing big questions about the future that
would come next, breaking the thread that bound us to the past. A rupture had been
created with the life lived up to that moment, and experiences of disorientation, loss,
nostalgia were prevalent, at least in the very early phase of the lockdown. Time was
suspended, ties to the past and future compromised.

I had recently started work at the University,[4] and the health emergency during
the lockdown period in Italy, from February to May 2020, had entailed the forced
blocking of in-person activities (classroom lectures) and in-company activities
(internships, etc.), unprecedented organizational changes (distance learning, suspension of services, online examinations), that added up to all the other changes
imposed on society to contain the spread of the virus, from isolation at home to the
suspension of all types of association activities.

When the period of tight lockdown ended I was attending a training experience
in Narrative Medicine, at Istud,[5] and it seemed natural, when we were asked to do a
project work using narrative methodology, to start collecting stories from the students enrolled in the Master's degree where I was supporting them for their internships, with the aim of understanding what impact the lockdown experience had on
their lives as young university students and more specifically on their well-being. I
prepared narrative diaries in which they could retrace those moments of the lockdown and testify through written narratives, photos, pictures, what their experience
had been. What came out was an intimate narrative that I would like to take back to
better illustrate the context in which we were living at that time.

In the stories collected there was a depiction of the initial time as pause-vacation,
along with a kind of self-distancing from what was happening. However, the

---

[4] I was in charge of coordinating curricular internship activities for the Master's degree program in
Human Resources Training and Development at Bicocca University in Milan.

[5] Istud is the first independent business school in Italy, based in Milan. ISTUD represents one of the
international references for the dissemination and application of narrative medicine. In 2016,
ISTUD served as a reviewer for the World Health Organization on how to apply narrative methods
in health care, "Cultural contexts of health: the use of narrative research in the health sector."

awareness of what was happening soon increased, and the emotional status changed with the experience of home isolation, media images (newspapers, TV), experiences of contact with the illness, and abrupt interruptions of daily projects and activities (internships, work, leisure, etc.). The emotional tone was mainly of fear and uncertainty. Asked to describe how they felt, the emotions reported were bewilderment, confusion, pensiveness, worry, dread, fear, anxiety, apprehension, and helplessness. Over time, the experiences of bewilderment and apprehension related to the pandemic became more pressing, more pronounced among students who were more exposed to the experience of the disease because they lived in the hardest-hit regions (Lombardy) or because they had suffered bereavements in their families. Time, emptied of daily routines and plans for the future, became an anxiogenic dimension, open to experiences of anxiety, worry, despondency.

In order to regain psychological well-being, the ability to establish a new routine, to scan the times of the day differently, relieving tension and sustaining a "do-as-if" strategy in search of a new normal, became essential. Hence, practices of yoga, cooking, or more generally linked to hobbies and interests became not only ways to occupy time, but strategies for a full rediscovery of oneself. The spread use of video conference systems on online platforms made it possible to meet the denied need for sociality and to feel less alone.

Nevertheless, a feeling of boredom, monotony of the days prevailed in the long run. Suffering from the experience of social isolation and the importance of a return to the normalcy of daily routine and social ties prevailed in many of the stories told. We had been deprived of our routines. We were all in the same boat, exposed to our existential loneliness.

> I feel it's a Salvador Dali painting that faithfully represents me, the stillness of a woman who looks out the window, to a boundless uncertain future, frightening and almost inaccessible, mixed with a sense of ill-concealed confidence that there is a place in the world for each of us in the end (notes from a student's diary).

All the ambivalence associated with domestic space emerged in their diaries: on the one hand, being at home harkened back to family, an image of warmth and safe shelter; on the other hand, there was impatience for the lack of freedom of movement, experienced by many as a real imprisonment.

The same themes and experiences emerged in the dreams of the matrices during the lockdown. We were no longer used to experiencing space and time differently. We had gone from running at 100 km/h to standing still and motionless. The lack of the dynamic element was missing; it was a resumption of an almost primitive time that created anguish. We were all grappling with a dishabituation from daily routines and searching for new habits to fill the days.

It is interesting to note, going to the roots of the word, that Habit in Latin comes from the word Habitus and the verb Habere (in English to have): meaning a way of being, disposition of mind, appearance, and also "clothing," that is, everything we are used to have with us, to carry around with us continuously. The pandemic and the lockdown were somehow asking us to relieve ourselves of our clothes that were no longer suitable for the new scenario.

At the time, I was reading an interesting book by Matteo Meschiari called *Disabitare* (Dis-inhabiting), reflections on the evolution and transformations of domestic spaces, with an anthropological view. The author in his work suggests an anthropological reading on how domestic spaces have developed over time as a function of a relationship with the external space. In fact, he says, the human species has never lived in contact with the outside but rather in intermediate places, in between the closed and the open space, highlighting the importance of the relationship between indoor and outdoor spaces in defining the logic and meaning of living.

Looking out the window during the period of the tight lockdown, the feeling of estrangement was strong. The lockdown had disrupted not only the time rhythms we were used to, but also the spaces we could inhabit that defined our actions. Images of empty streets, without people or vehicles, represented a lunar landscape. The streets were so quiet that from the rather large fountain near my house, ducks could go undisturbed in singular walks on the roadway. The outdoors had become off-limits, except for what was allowed by the government's decree; for many, the window to the world had become the Internet, and time was punctuated by activities that took place in the intangible environment of the Net. How much this new world, characterized by new ways of living space and time, was affecting us? What new habits would make more functional?

Dating back 15,000 years is the supporting structure of an Upper Paleolithic hunter's hut discovered in Mezhyrich Village, Ukraine in 1965. That complex bears the primitive traces of the practice of habitation where symbolic and functional aspects are combined in the logic of construction. At the entrance of the huts, built of mammoth bones, there was the presence of the skull of the animal itself, decorated with colored dots and lines of red pigment, interpreted as a stylized sign of fire. Much earlier, namely during the glacial period, it is assumed that Neanderthals did not live in real dwellings, but rather in natural shelters, inhabiting damp and cold caves: the space only served as a shelter from the external weather through rudimentary screens. Space, Meschiari says, became "home" the very moment symbolic thought appeared.

I found this quite enlightening. The interesting reflection coming from these studies on primitive shelters represents the closest link between habitation and symbolic capacity, also in reference to the value of alterity.

> Analyzing then the prehistoric forms of dwelling we notice essentially two things: the openness to the outside and the reference to animality (...). Other (animality) and Elsewhere (the landscape) are crucial elements of early dwelling, they are the identity/alterity device cast in the stem cell of man's spatial foundation. [10, p. 42]

Dwelling is thus not only related to a modification of space to respond to primary needs (finding shelter) but to the attribution of a symbolic meaning that is defined in relation to the outside, the animal part, the landscape. That is, there is an "extroverted" dimension of dwelling that led us to ask ourselves, thinking about inhabited places, using Meschiari's words, "Where is the animal? Where is the landscape in this house?"

The uninhabited space we were experiencing became even more of an interesting object of reflection in light of these studies on the emergence of the first dwellings.

Back to the lockdown, we were suddenly inside a new, alienating landscape that required reconfiguring the relationship between inside and outside. What had our homes become? Were we not, like our primitive ancestors, seeking refuge from the external threat of the looming pandemic? How were we experiencing this transformation of the landscape? What forms of "domestication" and symbolization were we deploying in order to inhabit the new landscapes that were before us?

It was during our team meeting after the first matrix that the word Habitat came to our minds. As we pointed out already, Habitat comes from the Latin "habitare," which in its proper sense means "to continue to have," but more commonly means "to have custom in a place," "to inhabit." In ecology, the term habitat refers to the place that possesses the most suitable physical and environmental characteristics that allow a given species to live, develop, and reproduce. Environment, social context, space, territory, fabric are synonyms.

These and other reflections were important cues for dealing with the material that emerged in our Social Dreaming experience during the lockdown. The sudden transformation of our natural habitat had made difficult to understand the connection with living inside home, in the domestic context and one's interiority. The symbolic dimension of dreams was a way to relate with the external context, processing the ongoing transformations of what was happening "outside" the home. Through the concept of Habitat, an attempt was made to capture this dynamic between the external and the internal world.

Each matrix therefore became the beginning of a quest for meanings. We transformed the dream sequences into images and tried to understand their dialogue with the external. The collection of images made for each Social Dreaming session, enclosed in a common frame, was called Habitat. The word Habitat seemed the right one to use for the new landscape at the time of the pandemic.

References

1. AA.VV. Argo. A modern story, beyond sailing. Asti: Hasta Edizioni; 2007.
2. Frank AW. The wounded storyteller. Chicago, IL: University of Chicago Press; 1995.
3. Baricco A. Quel che stavamo aspettando. Milano: Feltrinelli; 2021.
4. World Health Organization. Mental health and Covid 19: early evidence of the pandemic's impact. World Health Organization; 2022.
5. Margherita G. L'insieme Multistrato. Roma: Armando editore; 2012.
6. Bion W. Apprendere dall'esperienza. Roma: Armando editore; 1962.
7. Organisational and social dynamics. Oxfordshire: Phoenix Publishing House; 2021;21(2).
8. Organisational and social dynamics. Oxfordshire: Phoenix Publishing House; 2020;20(1).
9. Lingiardi V. Mindscapes. Milano: Raffaello Cortina Editori; 2017.
10. Meschiari M. Disabitare. Antropologie dello spazio domestico. Milano: Meltemi; 2018.

Chapter 3
Dreams at the Time of COVID-19: A Social Dreaming Experience

3.1 The Project of the 4 Social Dreaming Matrices: General Description

Gordon Lawrence, the creator of Social Dreaming, borrowed the term "matrix" from the German/British psychoanalyst S.H. Foulkes who described the group as a living organism, to enhance the characteristic of the Social Dreaming as "a space in which something happens."

It is important to point out that Gordon Lawrence conceived Social Dreaming as a generative space of new ideas of unexpected potential, a primordial space, a maternal womb that reminds to the common origins of humanity. In particular, Lawrence highlighted the difference between a group experience and a matrix experience, where the former focuses on the dynamics between the participants within the group, while the latter is a space of potential understanding that only happens in the absence of interpretation and judgment.

The Social Dreaming Matrix (from now on SDM) is a group meeting lasting about one and a half hours, which can be repeated at set intervals. The composition of the group can vary from a minimum of 12–15 people to a maximum of around 30, although matrices with a much larger composition can often be conducted.

If the meeting takes place in presence the participants to the matrix sit in a spiral in an arrangement called "snowflake-shaped," in order to avoid direct eye contact and facilitate the centering on a "middle space," partly internal and partly external, that favors the connection of one's inner emotions and the resonances with the others.

The sessions have a narrative unfolding, alternating the sharing of dreams with the free associations that emerge as they unfold.

The SDM is convened by a "host" (or more than one in the case of large groups), whose function is to "protect the boundaries" of the matrix, providing a safe container for everyone's free expression and to facilitate connections, highlighting the

E. Pasini, C. Trimboli, *A Social Dreaming Experience at the Time of COVID 19*,
New Paradigms in Healthcare, https://doi.org/10.1007/978-3-031-42498-4_3

links between the elements that appear in the matrix in the absence of judgment and interpretation that could block the free flow of associations.

What matters most therefore is "what the host does not do": does not interpret dreams in relation to the personality of the dreamer; does not saturate the possible meanings that develop in the matrix; stands in the "not knowing" position until a common pattern emerges, cultivating the "negative capability" to remain in uncertainty, mystery, and doubt, without turning to an impulsive search for facts and reasons.

At the start of the SDM the host recalls the primary task of the matrix with the ritual question "who wants to bring the first dream?"; emphasizes the importance of nonjudgmental listening, reminding the hope that everyone could "leave their ego outside the door" to enter a flow from which is possible to access to a dimension of potential discoveries.

At the end of the SDM, a set time (which length can vary from 15/30 min and more) is dedicated to the Dialogue Reflection Dream (DRD), in which participants begin to verbalize the experience of the matrix and question themselves about the dreams and their meaning. Like the moment of the waking up, the ego that had been momentarily set aside can now recover its thinking function, and the different patterns emerged in the matrix can be recognized, amplified, connected, in a network of correspondences.

The project of the Social Dreaming Matrices was held between mid-March and early May 2020 every 2 weeks, from the first week of lockdown on mid-March, to the end of the lockdown at the beginning of May. During this time 4 Social Dreaming sessions were held, on March 17th, April 1st, April 15th, May 5th 2020.

Each session lasted for about 2 h, from 6 PM to 8 PM CET, 1 h was devoted to the Dream Matrix, 45′ to the Reflection Group; each Matrix was followed by a staff members meeting.

The group of the participants was formed on a voluntary base, as a dreamlike exploration during the first lockdown in Italy; the "dream hunters" gradually increased in number from one session to the other, from 15 people at the beginning to up to 30 at the end. The group that gradually formed was mostly composed of professionals in the area of business consulting and training, psychologists and psychotherapists, researchers in marketing and social areas, university students, volunteers involved in social works.

The staff was composed by the host of the Matrix, one co-host and two coordinators, essential for the search and the treatment of the images and the creation of multimedia materials (short videos editing of film clips).

The 4 SDMs were held online in a Zoom platform. To create a dreamlike relaxing atmosphere that could allow the participants to better focus on dreams the image of a starry night sky was screened in the first part of the experience, devoted to the sharing of dreams. Participants were asked to freely and spontaneously share their dreams, with no self-presentations and interpretations. In the Reflection Group participants go back to the Zoom grid screen mode.

At the end of the experience of the 4 SDMs a large group meeting was held, on July 9th 2020, to discuss the suggestions of the landscape of dreams developed by the collection of images of the staff.

The journey we had made together led us to the discovery of an evocative, surprising, sometimes disturbing imagery, which we shared through the production of short mash-up videos inspired by the "stories" collected through the dreams, in order to highlight the collective meanings arisen from the SDMs.

The result was a landscape of the dream imagery through the creation of dream maps, one for each one of the four stages of the journey: we called them the Habitat of the Matrix.

The description of the experience of the 4 Social Dreaming Matrices that follows is aimed to suggest to the reader to retrace our path.

The dream narratives have been transformed into images evocative of the relationship between the outer world and the inner world at the time of the COVID-19.

3.2   The Tale of the Experience: A Framework for Reading

> The narrative is present in all times,
> in all places, in all societies;
> the narrative begins with the very history of humanity;
> it does not exist, has never existed,
> anywhere a people without narratives […]
> the tale is like life.
> Roland Barthes [1]

Social Dreaming matrices have from the very beginning revealed their narrative power through dreams offering interesting food for thought. Indeed, they seemed to offer an interesting meeting point between the individual point of view and a broader, collective view.

In the dreams there were all the elements that help create that suspension of disbelief and allow one to become fully immersed in the narrative, typical of movie scripts [2]. There was internal consistency, in the situations and characters, despite the presence of many fantastic and unrealistic aspects. The narrative was supported by detailed description of the settings, the plot structured, there was finally a strong emotional involvement and a sense of authenticity. The dreams were for all intents and purposes stories endowed with some meaning.

In addition, the dreams told bore obvious common patterns and recurrence of similar images and themes. The dreams brought individually not only seemed to tell us about small stories, with well-defined scenes, characters, actions. Looking at the collected corpus as a whole, from the very beginning we had realized that there was a connection between the dreamed elements, a "red thread" that seemed to contribute to the collective "meaning" of the moment experienced in the Social Dreaming session.

Moreover, there seemed to be a connection between the inner imagery evoked by the dreams and the external context. We noticed that a different theme emerged in each session. The evolution of context situations seemed to spill over into the sessions in part, as if it were a parallel world that followed the evolution of the reality experienced during the day. We had a strong impression that we had in our hands a "dense material" carrying several recurring elements, from the images evoked to the themes reported and the structures of the individual narratives. We wondered: what is the deeper meaning of it all? What are the dreams telling us about?

Thus emerged the idea that behind the narrative of individual dreams could be hidden the plot of a deeper narrative, that this originated in the traumatic experience related to the COVID-19 and that, although experienced by individuals, at the same time managed to transcend it to become a source of understanding of what was happening to us as a collective.

The discovery of such evocative, surprising, and sometimes disturbing imagery led us to initially produce short mash-up videos inspired by the "stories" collected through the dreams (to be shown to participants in the final meeting) in order to highlight the collective meanings that arose from the SDMs.

Moreover, we wondered if we could consider the rich research material as a text, coupling a semiotic reading with a symbolic-interpretive reading of the elements that emerged. The semiotic research highlighted collective patterns and socially shared codes, which were analyzed and amplified on their symbolic content. More specifically, we treated the images as if they were film sequences, and we analyzed the material using Semiotic approach and Jungian symbolism.

Taking notes of the dreams was very helpful to find a rhythm for the narrative and for the filming sequences that was as faithful as possible to the narrative brought in by the participants, with the awareness, however, that some kind of reductionism was almost inevitable. To reduce risk, we sequenced the images using the same temporal progression with which they were told.

The narratives of the dreams had a strong imaginative impact, all of them full of colors, situations, places as vivid as film sequences; amplification through the dream sequence of certain recurring themes and images had a nonlinear, circular, and recursive logic.

We collected and sequenced all the dreams, then we focused on the images, signs, symbols, and myths, on the recurrences that so powerfully emerged, grouping similar themes, symbols, colors, situations, etc. By arranging the material in a staff work, we gradually came to identify the key elements of the structure: themes, actions, characters, oppositions.

The work analysis on the material of the Social Dreaming Matrices was a kind of movement from the outside inward, that is, from the dreams told to the search for deeper meanings, referring to the semiotic approach. Jungian Analytical Psychology and an anthropological approach allowed us to enrich the analysis with the symbolic and archetypal dimension.

More specifically, we worked on four different levels of analysis.

- We analyzed at first the more "superficial" elements of the dreams: colors, signs, symbols, images, words, etc.
- At a second level we searched for the "discursive structures": characters, places, times of the tale, themes, and associated figures.
- At a third level we looked for the structure of the story, referred to as semi-narrative structures and archetypal level.
- Finally, the fourth and deeper level defined the oppositions of meaning, on which we assumed the very structure of the text was based.

The first part of the analysis was devoted to formal aspects. We focused on the visual dimension evoked in the dream narrative, and in particular, the first thing we focused on was the superficial part: the symbols, settings, shapes, objects, colors, signs and images, and keywords.

The amplifying effect of Social Dreaming seemed to have created powerful connections between one dream and another within the same matrix. Although not in direct succession, it was evident that there was a certain repetitiveness of imagery.

Moreover, the dream dimension seemed to be connected to the here and now of the moment of dreaming together. In fact, at a distance of time, the imagery seemed to follow an evolution. It changed the imagery of signs, symbols, colors and with them, also the nature of the story itself.

We then dwelt on the characters, places, and concrete objects that were brought into play in the different dreams. Who were the main characters in the dreamed scenes? What actions were they performing? Who were they with? Were there allies or enemies to fight? What kind of narrative register emerged? Comedy or dramatic? Which archetypes emerged?

We looked at the elements that gave sense to the action: who were the "heroes" occupying the dream scene? Who were the antagonists? What were the links between the different elements and what were the "valuables" that caused movement in the story? These questions helped to reconstruct the plot.

We have thus arrived at the deepest level of the story, the one from which the overall meaning flows, which is generally related to the conflict generated between two opposites (e.g., a story may tell the clash between Life and Death, between Good and Evil, between Nature and Culture).

One of the most relevant figures in the semiotic structure of discourse, upon Greimas, is the so-called semiotic square, which represents the contrasts in a graphic scheme and indicates the fundamental values underlying a narrative and the transformations that occur within it. It is thus that gives movement to the story. The use of the semiotic square was effective because, as we will see in the next pages, in all the matrices the juxtaposition of opposite poles of meaning always clearly emerged.

Once we had identified the main opposition (e.g., Wild versus Domestic in the first matrix) we positioned the scenes according to whether they belonged to one of the two poles, beginning to draw the coordinates of a sort of map. We worked first on the emerging pair of opposites and then focused on the elements that did not seem to fully adhere to any of the main categories, but still seemed to be related to them in some way. We analyzed the spontaneously evoked symbolic and mythical material, and this helped a lot in the systematization.

More specifically this helped us to put an order in the oneiric chaos, to build "maps" of the psychic landscape, which we called Habitat, that in each Matrix seemed to have a distinctive fil rouge, with symbols, signs, metaphors, emotional tones, able to give an overall coherence to the narrative.

The dream narratives have been transformed into images evocative of the relationship between the outer world and the inner world at the time of the COVID-19. The result was a landscape of the dream imagery through the creation of dream maps, one for each one of the four stages of the journey: we called them the Habitat of the Matrix.

The outcome of the analysis was a set of maps of the Habitat, as the psychic landscape described by each Matrix. The exploration of the Habitat was both the "imaginal" description of the conscious and unconscious forces playing at each moment in the collective unconscious, and the "fil rouge" unraveling the whole narrative.

The theorical and methodology framework in which we moved is the qualitative research methodology [3, 4]. This term refers to an approach using multiple theories, methods, and techniques of reference that is aimed at producing knowledge about a given phenomenon, located at a given historical moment. The modus operandi of this type of research differs from that of quantitative setting which is driven by the idea of measurement and sizing. Statistical models of data measurement are not used. There is no ambition to measure and control. Rather, it moves within a logic of explaining and understanding the operating patterns of a given phenomenon, which are not visible at first glance.

We will share in the next paragraph some research data of the feedbacks from the participants after the SDMs experience, but we would like before share some thoughts regarding the validity of the results obtained. We start from the awareness that it is not possible to look to the objectivity and replicability of experience as the yardstick and measure to assess how effective our work was. The experience made will remain a unique and unrepeatable moment, contextualized in a precise historical moment and aimed at better understanding what was happening at that moment.

Rather, we believe that the work done may respond, more consistently, to other criteria and in particular to the four parameters that Riessman [5] introduced to address the issue of validation of narrative research, as indicated below.

1. Plausibility: The interpretation must be reasonable and convincing.
2. Correspondence: It is desirable that the results of the analysis be returned to the subjects, so that they have the final say [6].
3. Consistency: The interpretation must show internal consistency, that is, the text must be organic, both for those who formulate it and for those who read it, and the different parts must not contradict each other.
4. Pragmatic use: It must provide the information that will make it possible to determine the reliability of the work by describing how interpretations were produced, making visible what was done, specifying how we made subsequent transformations, making primary data available to other researchers.

We hope in conclusion that the work has made a contribution in shedding light on what seemed opaque, in making sense of what seemed to have no meaning and what no one expected to happen [7].

The description of the experience of the four Social Dreaming Matrices that follows is aimed to suggest to the reader to retrace our path.

The following of this chapter provides insights of the dream materials, metaphors, connections, images of each one of the four SDMs as accurate as possible, as well as a brief description of the events that marked the social context at the time. It is not possible here to submit all the images collected, we can provide just a few of them as an example worked to highlight the functioning of the associative process and the amplification of the connections between words and images that allowed us to identify the specific Habitat of each matrix.

3.3   First Social Dreaming Matrix: 17th of March 2020 – Loss, the End of a Way of Life

3.3.1   The Socio-Political Context at the Time

The first lockdown in Italy began on March 9, 2020.

On that day, the whole country was declared "red zone" and the Prime Minister Giuseppe Conte announced on TV drastic measures to contain the pandemic.

"Our habits must change now, we must all give up something. We must do it now and we will only succeed if we adapt to stricter regulations," Giuseppe Conte[1] claimed in the first of a long series of "edicts," establishing a general obligation to limit all kind of movements as well as any traveling in the country outside one's area of residence.

"I stay at home" was the claim of the moment that suddenly swept away the normality of the daily life: no more office work, no more school for children and youngsters, the family life was forced in a couple of rooms, all gathered around a computer screen.

The pandemic had taken us by surprise and no one could imagine, back then, how long the enforced isolation would have lasted, and what could have happened next.

Long queues in front of the supermarket to hoard primary basic goods reminded of the wartime; episodes of solidarity between neighbors seamlessly alternated with menacing "hunts for the pest," the guilty one blamed for spreading the pandemic walking the dog without wearing a mask.

The metaphor of war was obsessively repeated and endlessly emphasized.

"We are fighting a war on the virus," said the French President Emmanuel Macron.

The enemy, however, was an invisible entity that lurked in the most banal and harmless daily routines, transforming in a threat everything that used to be the normal life.

Threats of contagion, anxieties, fears were palpable presences, that people tried to exorcise saying "we can make it" and "we will come out of it better".

However, along with those omens of doom, the idea that such catastrophe of biblical dimensions was not something temporary and transitory after which we would have returned to a "new normal" life, that could hopefully be even better than before, but was instead a signal coming from the deepest, the tip of an iceberg that concealed a profound change we had unconsciously expected for a long time to happen.

In the only half-safe refuge of the confinement at home, enduring such a prolonged contact with ourselves and our solitary thoughts revealed to be increasingly difficult.

However, together with the discomfort, the unexpected desire for a different sociability, for different forms of intimacy, slowly emerged.

The expectation of a change was in the air, along with the search for new ways to explore what was happening inside and outside us.

---

[1] Giuseppe Conte was the prime minister of the current government at the time of the lockdown.

3.3.2   The Inner World at March 17: Images from the Dreams

> I have a glass of wine in my hands, beautifully shining at light, when suddenly it crumbles before my eyes falling into pieces.
>
> I'm driving a shiny new yellow Lamborghini, I don't like much driving cars, I wonder if it's mine and why I'm driving it. I'm driving through narrow streets in a crowded city when the car starts to lose its pieces, I'm astonished.
>
> I dreamt of losing all my teeth, is a recurring dream I had many times in many difficult situations.
>
> I get a phone call from my parents, then I enter the kitchen of their house, around the kitchen table my parents sit with six more people, I don't know them, my father had spread a mountain of dried black figs on the table, they are all neatly arranged, I look at my mother's face, she has her eyes circled in black, the eyes look similar to the black figs.
>
> I relive the same scene several times, I am on the phone in my small apartment, then I walk out of my room to talk to my roommate, I hear the phone ringing again and re-enter my room, the same scene repeats two, three times, I feel a strong anxiety.
>
> I am at home, looking out of the window I can see a raven and a pigeon, they are much bigger than they used to be, I think is an omen that brings bad luck.
>
> A bird, it could be a crow, looks like a totemic entity, a deity with a bird's head.
>
> I see a big sun, I know is a godhead, a big crowd of people turn to him adoringly, enchanted by its rays, it makes me think to the god Ra of the Egyptians, the sun god with a bird's head.
>
> A huge parrot with a big yellow beak, it cannot fly, looks very menacing.

Many dreams evoked by participants seemed to refer on the one hand to violated everyday scenes and on the other to a world populated by threatening animals. This first block of dreams seemed to us to stage the opposition, in the imagination, of two conceptual categories: the domestic and the wilderness.

The images of the dreams of the first Social Dreaming Matrix on March 17th, one week after the starting of the first lockdown, evoke a reality that is falling apart in front of our eyes, in the unsettling scenario of an everyday life that, beyond all appearances, has nothing left of familiar. Confined indoors until further notice, the daily routine abruptly changed, the order of things unnaturally subverted, deprived of many of the usual relationships, we were living in a kind of suspended time.

Confined in a time-bubble facing into the unknown, the objects that used to be part of our daily life and usual habits suddenly seemed to acquire a menacing aspect. They were still within reach as usual, but what embodied before our reassuring normality had abruptly changed into mysterious, frightening, disturbing presences, that seemed to have, at the same time, something unavoidable and inexorable. A looming threat was creeping into what had previously provided a semblance of stability to a hectic life, and the reassuring domestic feeling of being at home, the comforting feeling of family intimacy, was suddenly revealing its hidden face. Like in a horror movie, disturbing shadows lurked in the home objects, beyond the apparent normality where we would have liked to find refuge, giving shape and substance to what Freud called the "Unheimliche," the Perturbant.

The images of the dreams featuring hitherto familiar people and situations—a phone call from the flatmate, the parents gathered around a kitchen table with dried figs on the top (see Fig. 3.1)—triggered a nameless anguish and a sense of estrangement that was increasingly difficult to bear. Indulging in the comforting idea of

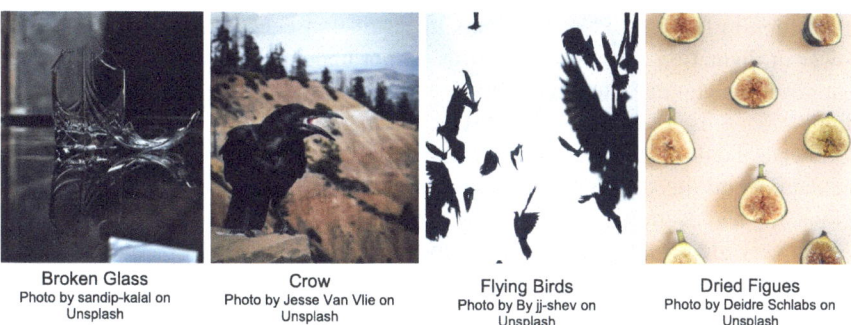

| Broken Glass | Crow | Flying Birds | Dried Figues |
| Photo by sandip-kalal on Unsplash | Photo by Jesse Van Vlie on Unsplash | Photo by By jj-shev on Unsplash | Photo by Deidre Schlabs on Unsplash |

Fig. 3.1 The images of the dreams depict a first pair of opposites, between Domestic and Wilderness

living on a threshold that sooner or later we would have find the way to cross, we were telling ourselves that this empty time would necessarily had to have a limit and therefore also a meaning. But we could not imagine how the world outside might have changed in the meantime, what we could find beyond the doorstep. In the "middle ground" at the border between reality and imagination, unexpected conflicting emotions were growing, that we were not at all prepared to bear: surprise, anxiety, astonishment, disquiet became the faithful companions of our days at home.

In a landscape deserted of humans, bird-headed deities reminding to the Egyptian sun gods Ra and Horus were showing up in the dreams. Huge parrots that could no longer fly, large pitch-black crows, like disturbing intimidating presences that were taking over in the urban territory we could grasp only small glimpses of them from the home windows (see Fig. 3.1). The images of a wild powerful nature counterpointed the deep feelings of being trapped, isolated in the domestic space. In the space outside an overwhelming world of unbridled instincts was taking over like in a kind of divine punishment, in front of which we felt helpless, at the mercy of a powerful nature (see Fig. 3.1). But if punishment refers to sin and guilt, were we punished for doing something wrong? And what did we do wrong? What was happening was our responsibility? Did we really deserve all this? Feeling of anger and despair were growing in the face of a punishment we did not believe we deserved.

The color yellow dominates the scene—yellow-beaked parrots, sun godheads, yellow Lamborghinis falling into pieces. The yellow is symbol of the sun, and of an absolute, transcendent, overwheling power. But at the same time, in China is the color of the imperial wisdom, hope and prosperity, sign of a process of transformation in motion. Wild natural elements and negative omens constellate the need for domestic safety, projections of strong emotions such as fear, sadness, loneliness, anger, which are too strong to bear and are therefore projected on the outside. But in the meantime the forced isolation obliges to look into themselves starting a process of introspection.

Birds appear in dreams as the main protagonists of the landscape outside, of all the animal species the one that has always mostly stimulated the human imagination. Since our ancient ancestors saw them soaring into the sky for the first time, their flight evoked the divine capacity to move from one element to another, connection to heaven and earth, embodiment of transcendence and of the arcane power of divination and prophecy. Birds do not undergo to the same natural laws that govern the human life; their flight represents a challenge to the laws of gravity, stimulates a sense of achievement, inspires divinatory arts, gives wings to imagination, feeds the desire for transcendence, reminding us of the possibilities of linking the natural and the supernatural realms, spirit and instincts, conscious and unconscious, life and death.

The very idea of transcendence is populated by winged figures: Aphrodite, the Greek goddess of love, is symbolized by a white dove, and the same is for the Holy Spirit of the Christian Trinity, the bearer of wisdom and light. Angels are winged figures, half birds and half humans, helping protective figures who mediate between heaven and earth. Hermes, the winged-footed Greek god herald of transformation, often in mythology plays the role of the psychopomp or "soul guide"—a conductor of souls into the afterlife. Apollo, the Greek god of divination and of the medical arts, had a raven as a messenger and companion, herald of misfortune but at the same time of the link between life and death, as we will see later in this chapter with the myth of Apollo and Coronides evoked by the matrix. Eventually it is important to emphasize that the large appearance of birds in the dreams reminds to the freedom of movement that we humans have lost is instead, for birds, within the grasp, the very essence of birds' life indeed, feeding the instinct that drives thousands of species of birds to migrate twice a year, northwards in spring and southwards in autumn, to lay their eggs, giving continuity to life. Their "migratory restlessness" sounds therefore a warning which has, at the same time, the sense of destiny, something that was once familiar and that we desperately miss today. Then there was a second group of emerging dreams that seemed instead to propose scenes of intimacy-seeking contrasted with a "frozen," interrupted external social space.

I am at an animated gathering full of people, all of them are very young, beautifully cheerful and smiling. They exchange glances and an intense current of eroticism fills the air. I am among them but feel estranged and isolated, I have the task to make a presentation but the time seems to be stuck, the presentation never starts, there is uncertainty about the timing, everyone asks me questions and I don't know what to say, I have no idea of what could happen, then I find out that there is another meeting in another place and I tell everyone they should go there.

Pile of shoe boxes are stacked on the edge of a window, rectangular, long, they look like small coffins. There are six boxes stacked one on top of the other in two groups of three, I open them all one at a time and find some old pairs of shoes I use to wear long time ago, they remind me of times gone by. But I know I don't need them now, I think they are not the right shoes. I stand on a stool to reach the boxes when I look at the window frame above me and realize that I am in the bathroom of the old seaside house of my childhood, in the small town of Cesenatico on the Italian Adriatic coast. Then I remember a game we used to play when we were children with my brother and my cousins, we went to the bathroom and locked the bathroom door from the inside, getting out from the small upper window above the toilet which was too little for an adult to pass through. The bathroom stay closed for hours, and the adults had to beg us for opening. I feel a sudden feeling of peace and containment.

I am in a domestic environment, a house I often see in my dreams, I'm standing in front of a large window, looking out I see an expanse of empty bar tables. The house inside looks like a gym, a very nice environment I think. I climb the stairs to go to the first floor, I'm

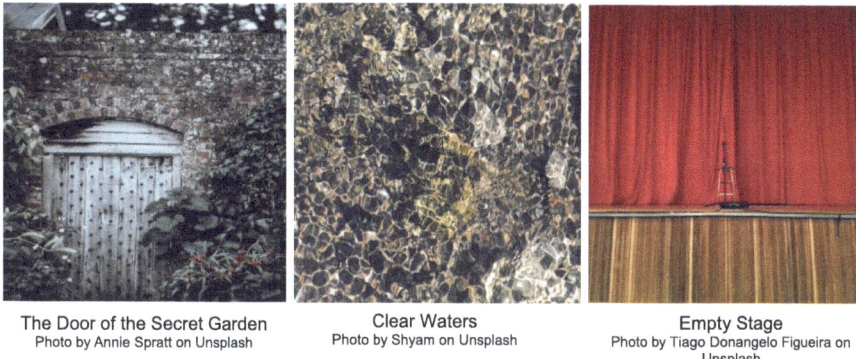

The Door of the Secret Garden
Photo by Annie Spratt on Unsplash

Clear Waters
Photo by Shyam on Unsplash

Empty Stage
Photo by Tiago Donangelo Figueira on Unsplash

Fig. 3.2   The images of the dreams depict a second pair of opposites, between Intimacy and Social Space

searching for a part of the house I know exists, but I can't find it anymore. Then I see a small door closed with a padlock, I manage to open it and find myself in a terrace that looks onto a beautiful secret garden. It is not what I was looking for, but nonetheless I feel a deep sense of nostalgia.

I often feel sleepy, it happens a lot these days at home, and I think of the dreamtime as if it were a beautiful, clear, fresh waters. Today I fear living in the daytime much more than the nightime.

The rupture between the outer and the inner world is complete, and in the dreams the gaze turns inward, were secret gardens and crystal-clear waters to draw upon are hidden (see Fig. 3.2), together with memories of the childhood that may help to cope with the stuck, meaningless situation of the present. The inner search of meanings sounds like a challenge to escape the absolute overwhelming power of which we are at the mercy. But the desire for renewal is still shrouded in mystery, only taking form in the imagination. We can therefore only guess the existence of a "hidden garden" of the intimacy, whose beauty arouses vague feelings of restlessness and awe. A timeless world brings back distant memories, which are incredibly attractive but deeply disorienting, widening the narrow boundaries of consciousness with glimpses of longing and nostalgia. The inner world we find in dreams, however, is a world that is also made of endless repetitions, piles of shoeboxes like small coffins that contain pairs of shoes we no longer need, missed presentations, doors that purposelessly open and close, and the truth is that we have no clue where all this may lead.

The landscape outside, that we could only see from the home windows, was motionless and empty, as if under a spell. The hectic pace of our lives that punctuated the days before the pandemic had suddenly vanished, any kind of activity in the social sphere blocked, we were the silent spectators of a motionless world (see Fig. 3.2).

In the frozen time of the never ending "groundhog days," closed doors hint at deep isolation and the loss of so many life chances. The intimacy with ourselves we experience in solitude reminds to the time of mourning, deep down we are aware of the need to pause in this suspended time before being ready to leave.

A closed door poses a question and represents a dilemma: should we open it or not? A closed door marks the boundary between the two separated worlds of the Domestic and the Wilderness. "Access forbidden" is the admonition in front of a closed door, which on one side sounds like a prohibition, and on the other side like a possibility to connect two separated dimensions. The image of the door represents the threshold between the inner and the outer world, between the known and the unknown, between sleeping time and wakefulness. The gate is the boundary of the lost Garden of Eden, forbidden to Adam and Eve after their disobedience to God's will. But beyond punishment, fear, and guilt, the crossing of the threshold of Eden brings to knowledge and self consciousness.

The image of the window, instead, represents an opening to the world, the only possible view we have now to snoop what is happening outside. The window embodies an urge to see beyond the gaze that stimulates imagination, and the thin line that separates the visible from the invisible reminds, paraphrasing Saint Exupery's Little Prince, that "the essential is invisible to the eyes." The window represents a boundary we can control, the opening and closing of the window's shutters allows light to enter and shields it with a curtain when the sun is too strong. The window recalls the need to protect ourselves from the burning light of the sun, marks the passage of time, separates the day from the night, gives a different rhythm to the existence, and reassures that tomorrow will be another day.

3.3.3 The Myth that Emerged from the Matrix: Apollo and Coronis

The powerful god Apollo, tells the myth, fell in love with the young and beautiful Coronis and, before leaving her for a while to pursue his god affairs, asked his faithful servant the raven to watch over the maiden. The raven was at that time a bird with a beautiful snow-white plumage, and faithfully obeyed his master's will. When Coronis fell in love and betrayed Apollo with the young Ischis then, the raven immediately flew to warn the god about her betrayal.

Apollo, seized by anger, killed Coronis stabbing her with an arrow.

Before dying, however, Coronis revealed Apollo she was pregnant with his son and, because of his anger, he would have died with her. Repentant for his gestures, Apollo tried to bring Coronis back to life without success, but before posing her on the pyre pulled the baby out of his belly and gave him to the centaur Chiron to raise. The child was named Asclepius, inherited his father's curative gifts and became later the god of Medicine.

Apollo's anger however did not spare the raven, guilty of being the cause of Coronis' death, and the god changed the color of its plumage from white to black. "Too much talkative was the raven, which is why he suddenly saw his feathers blacken", Ovidio wrote.

What were the dreams of this first matrix telling us? What narrative was being enacted? Activated reflection led us to the myth of Apollo and Coronides, as we will try to explain below.

The myth of Apollo and Coronis speaks of betrayal, anger, loss, repentance, all strong and conflicting emotions that plunged Apollo into despair. The black color of the raven's feathers evokes those dark feelings of all, which is why the raven has been considered the herald of misfortune ever since.

Apollo is the god of clarity of conscience and intellect, the archetype of a harmonious, ordered world where the rational mind always prevails over the laws of chaos.

In the Apollonian world there is no room for disorder and chaos, but there is not much space for the vital force of feelings either.

The myth, however, tells a different story: because of the betrayal of his unfaithful lover Apollo is seized by anger, but soon afterwards repents of the violence of his wrath. Coronis' betrayal is a deep wound to the god's pride, undermines his image and clouds his mind, but also brings out the power of the emotions and the limits of rational control over them. Overwhelmed by anger, the Apollonian world shatters in pieces, like the glasses that shattered in hands in dreams. However, the myth also suggests that it is through the painful experience of loss that new hope may arise. Asclepius the healer, the son of Apollo, generated by the dying Coronis, ushers the possibility of the cure; he is raised by the centaur Chiron, "the Wounded Healer," the one who was wounded twice by his own arrow and each time succeeded on transforming the wounds into inner strengths. Which is why Chiron was taken by Jung as the symbol of introversion in analysis: turning the gaze on the inside, in fact, might start a process of self-healing capable of restoring the vital strength of the unconscious.

The betrayal of Coronis (in which the name of the Corona virus echoes) constellates the archetype of the Wounded Healer, suggesting the possibility that the disease would eventually lead to restore an inner self-healing power. Coronis and the raven counterpoint in the process one to the other, both the bearers of revelations that eventually reconcile their destinies in a dynamic process of destruction and rebirth. Their re-union highlights the deep connection between the art of medicine, the treatment, and cure, symbolized by Asclepius, and the art of divination, black magic, and death, embodied in the popular tradition by the raven.

During the big infamous plague of the sixteenth century the doctors wore raven-shaped masks to avoid contagion when visiting the sicks (see Fig. 3.3).

Fig. 3.3 The plague doctor's dress

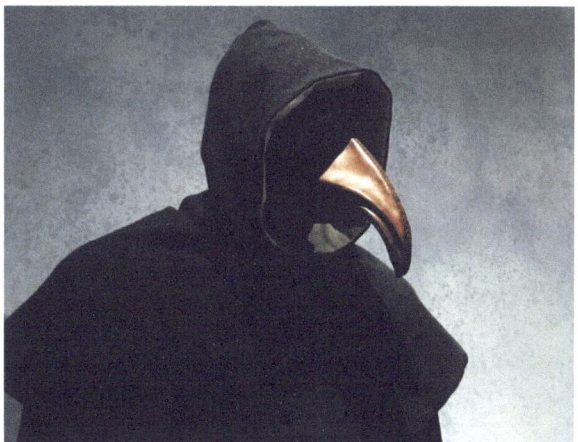

The plague doctor's dress refers to the clothing once used by doctors to protect themselves from epidemics. The dress consisted of a sort of black cassock long up to the ankles, a pair of gloves, a pair of shoes, a cane, a wide-brimmed hat and a beak-shaped mask containing aromatic essences and straw, which acted as a filter. (Wikipedia)

The similarities with the images of the medical and paramedical staff caring the COVID patients in intensive units is almost inevitable.

Through the sharing of dreams at the end of the first matrix the meaningless repetition of all-the-same days seemed to be more endurable, as if the exchange of dreams could transform the threatening signals of the unconscious into "clear, fresh, sweet waters." Overturning the relationship between conscious and unconscious, between the order of the day and the order of the night, the time of sleeping and of loss of consciousness seemed to be more comfortable than living in the waking time, where we were confronted with a reality that was too difficult to cope with.

3.3.4 The Habitat of the First Matrix

As anticipated, the tool used to visualize the new space that was taking shape, as a result of the solicitations from the external context, and the relationships between the symbolic categories that spontaneously emerged with the imaginary of dreams, is the Habitat. It is a kind of map, designed to respond to the need to organize in a frame of meaning what was collected and to synthetically represent the insights that arose during the matrix.

To resume the findings of the first SDM we would like to point out that from the dreams images emerge the relationship between the Outer world and the Inner world is played out on two pairs of opposites: Domestic versus Wilderness and Intimacy versus Social Space. The two opposition depicted in the chart below describe the first Habitat (see Fig. 3.4). The images in Fig. 3.4[2] are part of the imaginary dreamed and evoke the two pairs of opposites.

Opposition Between Domestic and Wilderness The first pair of opposites, the *Domestic* space of the house in which we are confined, and the *Wilderness*, the outside world to which we have no longer access, are two opposite, irreducible dimensions, impossible to hold together. Since the beginning of the lockdown we are living in a suspended time that is neither present nor future and evokes many ghosts of the past. In this altered dimension the objects of the house suddenly acquire some threatening, disturbing aspects. In the meantime the world outside has become a foreign dimension governed by natural forces, greater than ourselves. The overwhelming power of nature is represented in dreams by the birds we can spot from the house-windows, their flying high in the sky evoking transcendence and the power of the divine.

---

[2] Photos by Ken Batiov (Domestic), David Clode (Wilderness), Paolo Chiabrando (Intimacy), Karl Solano (Social Space) on Unsplash.

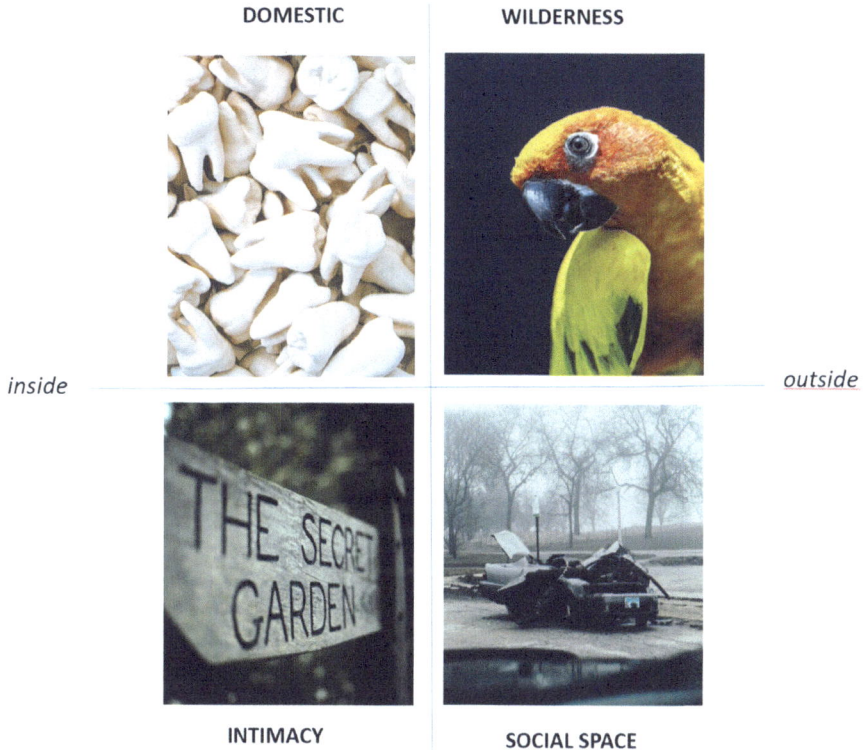

Fig. 3.4   Habitat of the 17th of March 2020

Opposition Between Intimacy and Social Space   The second pair of opposites, *Intimacy* and *Social Space*, highlights the theme of the threshold, which is at the same time a protection from a danger and a prohibition of crossing a boundary. In dreams we search for the "secret inner gardens of intimacy" that we believe we have lost, because the shattered, disconnected external reality is too hard to deal with. The relationship between the conscious and unconscious realms, between the order of day and the order of the night, is turned upside down; sleeping, the loss of consciousness, abandonment, seem more comfortable than the waking time.

3.3.5   Key Points of the First Matrix

- Domestic and Wilderness are opposite dimensions impossible to keep together.
- Intimacy and Social Space remind to a splitting and a separation from the instincts.
- Birds symbolize transcendence, the connection between earth and sky.
- The uncanny is embedded in the household objects.
- The emerging of the collective trauma: we live in a frozen time, "groundhog days" as meaningless repetition of the same pattern.

Key emerging question:
Is the garden of Eden irreducibly lost?

3.4   Second Social Dreaming Matrix: 1st of April 2020 – Bewilderment: The Search for a New Balance

3.4.1   The Socio-Political Context at the Time

At the beginning of April 2020 the restrictions of personal freedom increased exponentially along with the virus curve. The weekly "edicts" of the Prime Minister Giuseppe Conte announced further random measures of the virus containment, involving more severe restrictions of the freedom of movement: traveling within the country was forbidden except for exceptional certified needs; gatherings in public places were totally prohibited; shops, bars, restaurants, cinemas, and theaters had to remain closed until further notice; any kind of work that was not of public utility was allowed only on remote, as well as all classes and all kind of educational activities in schools and universities; trains, planes, extra-urban public transports were suspended, in the cities few bus lines worked with severe restrictions and compulsory sanitation; any connection with foreign countries was interrupted; finally, any violation of rules was considered a criminal offense, punished with severe fines and even the imprisonment in the most serious cases.

The confinement at home gradually became daily routine. To relieve the discomfort people invented new habits, made plans to share the home space between the family members, set up all sorts of online meetings to catch up on social life with distant relatives and friends, took lessons of cooking together and yoga in the living room. In such a highly critical situation,feelings of inequalities and discrimination increased among the population, between the lucky few who had comfortable houses, huge gardens and terraces at their disposal and the majority of the families that were obliged to share the space in small flats. In addition, a concern increased for the frailest, elderlies and children, not self-sufficient and more exposed to the contagion. The few acts of rebellion were harshly stigmatized in the media by the public opinion: *"A country united against Covid,"* headlined one of the major newspaper, pointing out that 3 out of 4 citizens described the atmosphere in the families as positive, 90% of citizens considered the measures against the pandemic very helpful, 89% thought they were clear and effective. The trust on the medical and paramedical staff and the Civil Defense that stood at the front line in the fight against the virus reached the highest scores. Experts, doctors, virologists of all kind and disciplines were omnipresent in the national TV.

Meanwhile, in the outside, the urban space previously occupied by man seemed now to be totally at the mercy of nature: roe deer and fawns invaded the streets, wolves returned to the cities, pigeons nested in empty nurseries; the human presence seemed to have disappeared from the scene, and the nature was quickly taking over in revenge.

The fear of the irreversibility of the change had turned into a growing anxiety about the future, and the long-awaited desire for a return to the old life now seemed far from being possible, taken for granted, perhaps even desirable. The future ahead was clouded with uncertainties, putting a strain to the longed-for search for a new balance. Moreover, an obsessive media campaign turned the need for guidance and support into the dangerous feeling of being trapped in a prison from which it would be increasingly difficult to escape.

3.4.2 The Inner World at April 1st: Images from the Dreams

I'm at home, in my bedroom, in front of a mirror. Two cats stare at me in amazement as I search the right dress to wear.

I enter a library that looks like a greenhouse, two people are talking to each other, unaware of my presence, the books on the shells are completely covered by lushing plants, the all ambience is suffocating.

I am in a Peruvian shop, full of beautiful jewelry, I spot a little girl who is wearing a necklace with a beautiful stone that is too big for her.

I open a drawer at home and I find by chance two beautiful necklaces I bought years ago, they bring back old memories, stories of travels I did long time ago in faraway countries.

I am on a terrace surrounded by walls decorated with ancient bas-reliefs, the place could be ancient Jordan city of Petra. A cat is scratching the sand and the beautiful bas-reliefs disappear before my eyes, only grains of sand remain. I stand motionless in disbelief, doing nothing.

I am in a garden in front of an ancient column, above which is the figure of a caryatid, I don't dare to get close and only take a picture from distance.

I am wandering around in a casbah in Jerusalem, with me four people I know, suddenly I realise that one of them has stolen my camera.

I am swimming underwater between mangroves and roots that turn to mush, a big mouth swims towards me but I am not afraid of it, this is life, I tell myself.

After one month of isolation the outside world has taken on phantasmatic dimensions. In a first group of dreams nature has definitively taken over, prevailing over culture (see Fig. 3.5). In the dreams we find ourselves crossing landscapes reminiscent of familiar sensations, but with bizarre unrelated aspects.

The number two recurs in the dreams (two cats, two necklaces, two colors...), highlighting feelings of separation and distance, but also the opposite, a deep desire for reunion and bonding. Symbolically, the number 2 is feminine, passive, receptive. In the I-Ching the number 2 represents the Yin principle, which is linked to the magnetism of the Earth, in opposition to the number one, masculine, that represents the dynamism of the Yang. The number 2 refers to the polarity between the masculine and the feminine, suggests the possibility of their re-union, is the number of the

Fig. 3.5 Library
surrounded by Ivy

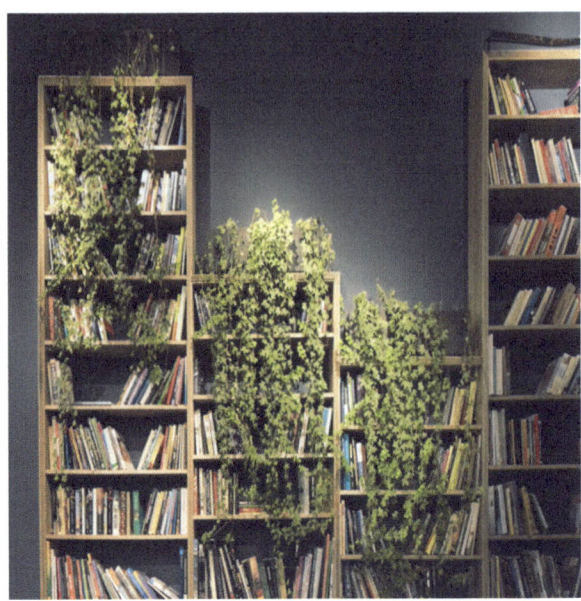

couple, of intimacy and harmony. But the number 2 also conceals a block, being stuck in a situation, the tendency to avoid conflict, to the point of passively adhering to the immutable laws of nature.

Culture instead appears in many dreamlike scenes in its collective, historical side. Images of the most beautiful monuments of ancient civilizations are threatened by a looming nature that strives to take back the spaces that men have conquered over the centuries. Man's dominion over nature has been overturned and the natural forces circulate unleashed without control. The archaeology of the past, the most beautiful artifacts of the human culture, are in danger to be annihilated, wiped out by a nature that erases the traces of the human race.

The cultural sites that appear in the dreams—Petra, Jerusalem, cities of the Italian Renaissance, caryatids—are powerful representations of the collective cultural imaginary, embodying an ordered familiar world made of shared rules and values that were part of a common history. A reassuring image of traditions capable of lasting on time. This important heritage of the past, however, is now threatened of disappearance by the scratch of a small cat. The entire human culture, all the customs and traditions based on experience and a collective history passed on from generation to generation, is at stake, and the fear of losing them makes us despair.

Meanwhile, another group of dreams emerged that seemed tense to represent the contrast between the disorienting and uncomfortable outside world and the ambivalent search for places in which to take shelter.

> I am at the opening of a new club, in the middle of the crowd a handsome young man stares at me insistently, the song The Prisoners played by the Italian singer Caparezza fills the air.

I'm chatting in Whatsapp with the Prime Minister Giuseppe Conte, then we are together in a room, alone, he speaks to me in a friendly quiet tone, he tells me "I'm going out this evening, if you want you could do it too".

I'm walking in the street at early morning, passing through a coffee shop full of people drinking coffee, I think this is not right, is prohibited, I'm scared. Then I get into the underground, it's full of people that are swimming in shallow water, all of them are dressing colored swimming caps, tapping hands and feet repeatedly in the pavement.

I have a therapy session with a patient but I can't find the right clothes to wear, many people come in the room all at once together with my patient but I am not ready for the session.

I'm half-naked in the midst of a group of people, I am wearing only a pair of trousers, suddenly all of them start laughing and I realize the trousers are not mine but my partner trosers.

A boundless beach is running parallel to a motorway, I'm walking side by side with my mother and a child, on the one side there are deep woods, in which I spot a man hiding to exercise, on the other side I see many people taking bath in pools of water in the middle of the woods.

Two frightening colors, yellow and purple, suddenly appear on my mobile phone to mark the rising curve of the virus, I'm got by panic.

I am in a conference room full of people, next to me is my wife, she does not speak English, I'm concerned but I can't see the speaker coming, I'm wondering where he could be.

I am in my hometown in the Marche region of Italy, at a running competition, I like running and I am good at it. Next to me there is a very slow runner but I cannot overtake him, I feel deceived, helplessness, I can't move.

I am in the van of my old theatre group, with whom I used to perform many years ago. We drove with the van from one show to another, it was a very special vintage car filled with many peculiar objects, that were for me precious memories of that time, now I see they are still there, I would like to take some of them with me but I can't, I have to leave them behind.

Looking out of the window in my house I see a beautiful, snow-covered mountain landscape. Someone is ski-touring on a slope of fresh snow, it could be me, the skis trace an invisible line on the soft snow at my knees. Suddenly I am seized by a deep feeling of great sadness because the all scene reminds me the death of a close friend.

Dreams depict a world we do not recognize, in which we do not know how to move. We walk on empty highways winding through forests of trees and deserted beaches; the underground is filled with water like a swimming pool; we cannot find the right clothes to wear, cannot run as fast as we used to. The surreal landscape is like an apocalyptic scenario, reminiscent of the dystopian worlds described in many movies—we mention *I'm a Legend* with Will Smith, in which the human race is destroyed by a virus and the cities are populated only by zombies—memento of biblical disasters like the Noah's ark and the big flood that submerged the world.

The once familiar landscape is now an estranged land in which we struggle to move. Any point of reference has blown away, we feel awkward and clumsy walking through the streets of our city.

In this apocalyptic scenario the dimension of power has lost its characteristics of an absolute divine force that had in the previous matrix. On March 17, at the beginning of the lockdown, the power appeared in the dreams founded on tablets of law that cannot be transgressed. However, was also an almighty powerful guide that could be trusted and relied upon. Now the dimension of power is instead elusive and contradictory —Conte, the head of the Italian government, tells in private "you can get out if you want" in a confidential tone—; an empty power expressed through purposeless edicts, a vexatious power that must be obeyed for no reason—the Caparezza's song The Prisoners speaks of a harsh prison and a pointlessly coercive power, the leit motiv of the song is "end of sentence never." Culture and power are empty spaces, meaningless, out of context dimensions.

What we described on March 17 the "uncanny domestic" has become now a disorienting space, in danger of being about to disappear, in which people struggle to find protection. Two opposites, fear of Chaos and need for Shelter, point to highlight an overturn of rules between Nature and Culture, in a hostile Habitat where the survival of the human beauty, history, and heritage is at serious stake. In this impossible environment we feel awkward, inadequate, powerless, unable to react. We feel we are out of place, bewildered. But is this because our fault, or are others who are barbarians?

The inner experience brought to light by dreams is very different from a fortnight ago. Walking in the outside is full of dangers, we seek refuge in small spaces, in which we find shelter. At home we find by chance in wardrobes and drawers long-forgotten items, precious jewels memories of the past. We feel we are living in a stalemate, struggling to find a balance between conflicting emotions and desires. We mourn the loss of a secure world and feel strong pangs of panic of an unnamed anguish. When we know the danger we have to fight fear is a warning bell that help to prevent the damage. Now, however, we feel harmless against unknown dangers lurking from every corners, threatening us and quickly taking over. Locked at home in a timeless confinement, we feel like prisoners in jail at the mercy of an unnecessary coercive power. The intimate, nostalgic mood of our wandering around in the house highlights the wish to find protection in the happy memories of the past, banishing the threatening thoughts of death and loss that constantly accompany us.

Trapped in a prison from which we cannot escape, similar to the one that was evoked in the matrix by the Caparezza's song. The prisoner, we feel pangs of the energetic charge of rebellion. The soft protection of the shells, the puddles of water along the motorways, the old vans, the stories hidden in necklaces and jewellery, that counterpoint the dreams relieve the harshness of reality, trying to make it more bearable (see Fig. 3.6).

The recovery of the memory of a happy past is like an intimate journey. The comforting objects found by chance, however, are also memories of what we have lost, and the precious necklaces suddenly turn out to be nooses tightened around the neck, the cherished van recalls the Noah's ark that saved few humans and animals from the flood.

The nature outside offers only a solitary comfort and a temporary shelter: hiding in the forest to exercise, bathing in puddles of water in the middle of the woods, walking through the yards of abandoned highways covered by grass, is not relief for the widespread sense of animpending danger lurking everywhere.

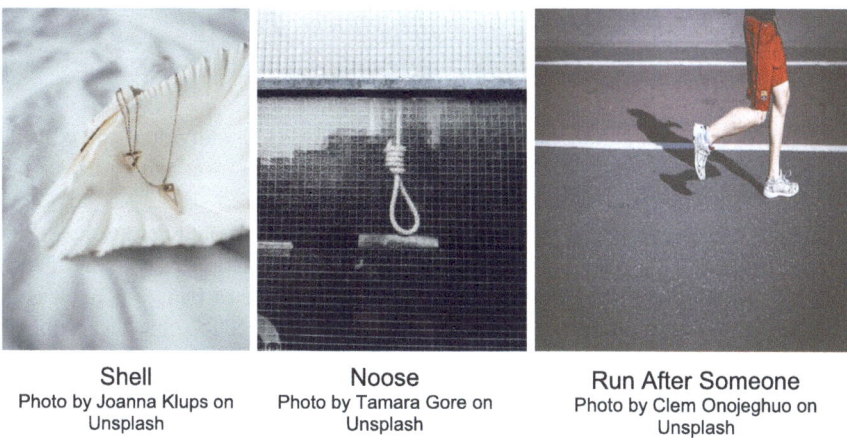

Shell	Noose	Run After Someone
Photo by Joanna Klups on Unsplash	Photo by Tamara Gore on Unsplash	Photo by Clem Onojeghuo on Unsplash

Fig. 3.6 Dreams from the imaginary, between chaos and shelter

Two emotional dimensions play against each other. On the one side the feeling of being trapped in jail, which is full of the energy of rebellion. On the other side comforting memories of the past acquire a nostalgic flair, concealing death and loss.

The secret garden of March 17, that represented an internal space of intimate discovery foreshadowing a possible expansion of the self, embodies now the struggle of the ego to protect itself from the troubles of the external world. The small precious objects scattered all along the way represent the splitting of the ego, longing for a comfort zone as a refuge against bewilderment.

To reconcile this splitting, was raised the connection with the work of the anthropologist Bronislaw Malinowsky, who in his book the *Argonauts of the Western Pacific* describes the circuit of the "kula," a form of ritual exchange practiced by the inhabitants of the Trobriands islands in the Western Guinea. Kula, says Malinowsky, means to go, and the kula circuit was the most arduous undertaking for the Trobriand's islanders. Embarked on fragile canoes, they periodically ventured into the open sea, following a predetermined route, only to bring precious shell necklaces and mother-of-pearl jewelry as a gift to strangers from other distant islands. The necklaces traveled clockwise, the jewels in the opposite direction, counterclockwise, and the only purpose that pushed the islanders to face such a dangerous journey was to make alliances, tighten relationships, consolidate economic power. Each object that entered the kula had a story, the story of the owner, whose deeds and prestige were handed down from hand to hand for ages. "Once in the kula, forever in the kula," the legend says, because in this kind of symbolic exchange objects embodied stories, alliances, relationships. They were therefore "good for thought", collective elements of a system of meanings that linked personal destinies and social order, beyond generations.

3.4.3   The Myth Emergent from the Matrix: Pan, the Theriomorphic God

The ruptures between Nature and Culture, Order and Chaos, individual and collective, conceals an irreconcilable archetypal contrast between Power and Order on the one side and the realm of Mother Nature on the other side.

The fears triggered by the pandemic made us feel helpless and defenseless. We have being caught by panic, because of our fragility. But is at this very moment, when all seems to be lost, that the long time forgotten voice of Pan, the Greek god of nature, resonates loud and strong. The prefix "pan" in Greek means "everything, keeping together". In times of chaos and despair, the voice of Pan is the last chance we have to overcome the deepest fears and the worst nightmares.

> In Greek mythology Pan is the god of Nature, and his origin is the Arcadia, which geographically corresponds to the today's Peloponnese, which has always been described as an idealized world where men and nature lived in perfect harmony. Bucolic poetry, from Virgil to the Italian Renaissance and Romanticism, made of Arcadia a place whose geography is rather psychic than physical. Pan, a multiform and ubiquitous god, can be found everywhere in caves, ravines, springs, woods and wild places, whenever instincts and desires meet. Always surrounded by nymphs who admire his sexual abilities, many lovers have been attributed to Pan, but no woman, nymph or goddess truly belonged to him.
>
> Pan the multiform god of uncertain birth, the son of many mothers and many fathers but ultimately loved by none. Pan the cherished child of the Olympus' gods and goddesses, mocked for his monstrous appearance and ultimately abandoned by all. Pan the vagabond, revered by shepherds and hunters, the theriomorphic god with goat feet, because of which was often associated with the devil. Pan the ubiquitous and the invisible, lighter than the air, who can suddenly appear and just as suddenly disappear. Pan, who is always associated with nightmares, with the power of the instincts, and madness. What could this peculiar and paradoxical god teach us today? When Psyche in her love torment for the young god Eros was seized with despair and attempted suicide by throwing herself into the river, Pan rescued her from the waters and gently placed her on the shore. Could Pan, today, be such a helping figure to us?

In his *Essay on Pan*, Hillman points out some important leads which is worthing to mention here. In the first place, Hillman suggests, Pan's close connection with the instinctual world reminds us that Nature is not something "outside of us" that speaks with a language we cannot understand, but is "inside of us," in all the sudden, instinctive reactions, which we put into action in some situations. The nameless fears we desperately try to avoid could therefore be, on a closer regard, a source of strength if they make us feel in deep connection with the natural world. The drive of instincts in fact means realizing that we are not irremediably separated from nature, but that we are actually part of it, that nature is part of our deep intimacy. Such deep awareness may represent today a source of hope when we are lost in despair.

Second, the language of nature is a language of images rather than abstract thinking. The same language of images that Jung placed as the foundation of the psyche and at the source of the archetypes, underlining that the psychology of the depth should move away from abstract concepts, rediscovering a "sensitive language," in order to get closer to the expressive power of the imaginal world. The death of Pan enshrines the loss of the creative language of nature, deprived of its generative capacity. Relying on our natural instincts may be sometimes dreadfully disturbing, but is nonetheless an essential part of an ontological experience which is today more important than ever.

Third, Hillman eventually says that "panic and paranoia can reveal an inverse proportion" [8], that the cause of panic is also the "royal road" that can dismantle paranoid defenses. This is "the therapeutic way to fear," when the existence is experienced through one's own instinctual vitality. When we are paralyzed by fear, the imaginal acquires an irresistible vitality, since we are connected to it through the instincts. What contains the nightmare and leads to madness can therefore also free us from it. Pan could therefore be the imaginal configuration of an instinctual world that acts as a bridge with nature, preventing psyche and nature from the split into two disconnected realities, on the one hand a soulless nature, on the other a soul without nature, psyche and matter irremediably separated.

Taking these reflections to their extreme consequences, we could say that the image of Pan is hidden today, in this time of pandemic, under our worst nightmares, fears, senseless events, nameless anxieties. Panic hides in the dark, behind what we have no explanations and answers. But the very fact that darknesses are ruled by Pan gives meaning and direction to chaos, and relief from blind actions without perspective. To make this happen, however, we should give space to intuition, the inner insights and sensory perceptions banished for too long. We should give up to the idea of a monocentric one-sided model of reality to recover a dialogue with a polycentric panel of images that still lives in us, even if through our worst nightmares.

3.4.4 The Habitat of the Second Matrix

From the dream images, it emerges that the relationship between the outer world and the inner world is played out in two pairs of opposition, Culture versus Nature and Shelter versus Chaos, depicted in the second Habitat (see Fig. 3.7). Images in Fig. 3.7[3] are part of the figures and characters emerged in the dreams and evoke the two pairs of opposites.

Opposition Between Nature and Culture The archaeology of the past, the most beautiful artifacts of human culture, are swallowed up by a powerful nature that is rapidly taking over, erasing all traces of the human race. A cat scratches the bas-reliefs of Petra turning them into sand, empty highways wind their way through deep forests and deserted beaches, wolves, pigeons, fawns conquer the space of cities.

---

[3] Photos by Jorge Fernández Salas (Culture), Maria Teneva (Nature), Noah S (Shelter), Becca Mchaffie (Chaos) on Unsplash.

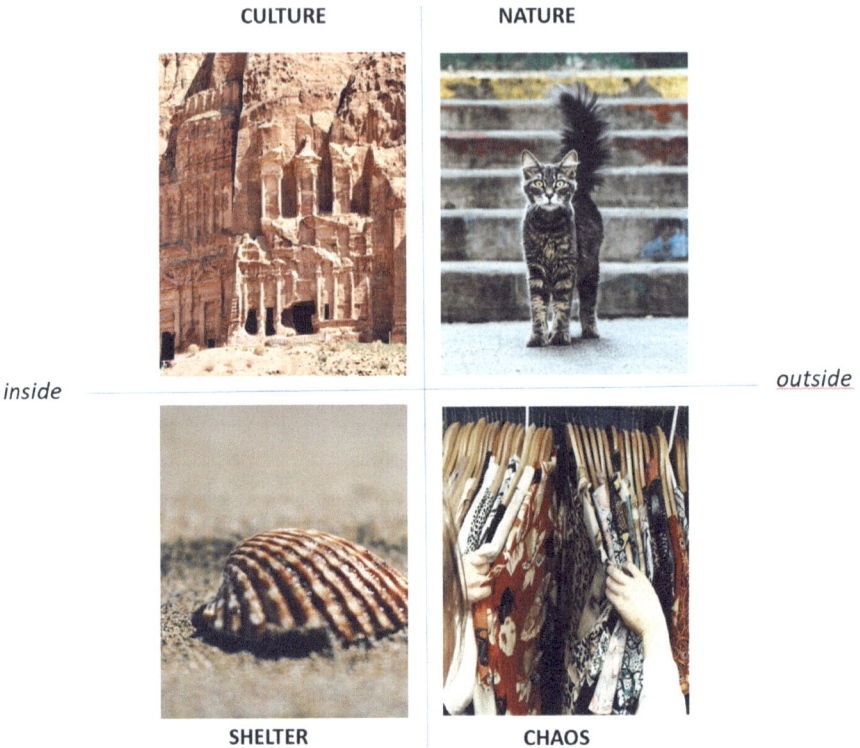

Fig. 3.7 Habitat of April 1st 2020

Opposition Between Chaos and Shelter On the outside, the order of things is subverted, the outer world is chaotic, disorienting, surreal, a world we do not recognize. On the outside we feel awkward and clumsy, meeting people in the street makes us uncomfortable, we seek shelter in small spaces, in which we feel imprisoned. Small treasures found by chance recall happy memories of the past and childhood.

3.4.5   Key Points of the Second Matrix

- Nature and Culture: The natural world prevails erasing trace of the human culture.
- Shelter and Chaos: The world outside is chaotic, we are seeking for repair.
- Feeling trapped in jail, for no reason, by an overwhelming power.
- Memories of the past are comforting and binding at the same time.

The key emerging question:

Should we stay or should we go?

3.5   Third Social Dreaming Matrix: 15th of April 2020 – Getting Lost in a Brave New World

3.5.1   *The Socio-Political Context at the Time*

More than 1 month has passed since the starting of the lockdown and the virus' growth curve has slowly started to decrease. In Italy the situation of the country, however, is a patchwork of differences region-by-region. In Lombardy the alert is at its highest, the situation remains critical and the intensive care units of the hospitals are still under highest pressure.

Easter and the summer holidays approach, and since the economy of many areas in Italy is based on tourism many regions show signs of discontent for the unlimited extension of the lockdown. The end was set for the beginning of May, but local authorities claim autonomy in their territory and local administrations try to gain power of decision over the central government, fueling internal disputes.

Growing doubts that the virus could be a gigantic maneuver hatched by subterranean powers to control the private lives of citizens and suppress basic freedom scattered among the people. Tempers were running high in endless exhausting discussions about the effectiveness of the measures that had been taken. The initially small group of "deniers" of the very existence of the virus was quickly growing in number, their protest and discontent making its voice heard loud. The idea that the pandemic was the result of a gigantic subterranean plot of the multinational economic and political lobbies, to control the private lives of the ordinary citizens acquired many followers in lower strata of the population, that were the most affected by the binding measures of containment and who feared the loss of economic livelihood more than the spread of the virus.

Freedom, citizenship, collective solidarity, the basic concepts that underlie a democratic state, seemed to have lost their social value, identified now in public debates only with the free accessibility to consumer goods and entertainment, anything that could be quickly obtained and quickly consumed.

The deniers of the pandemic targeted the excessive power of the pharmaceutical industry, pointing to the vast interests at stake in financing vaccine research and its production worldwide as the main principal cause of the massive spread of the virus. Social tensions increased. Meanwhile, the edicts of the central power became more stringent, detailed, complicated. Paranoid rules for the reopening made the day-to-day management of activities impossible for schools, hospitals, companies, public transport, shops, hotels. The lack of a clear understanding of what had to be done, what were the most important requirements for going back to the normal, where responsibilities should have been allocated, made increasingly difficult for citizens, companies, institutions to make decisions. Confusion reigned supreme. The desire to explore the new world after the lockdown was growing as much the worries about what we might find outside.

3.5.2 The Inner World at April 15 the Images from the Dreams

I'm playing at the Shanghai sticks, taking out the sticks one by one, I know that if I make a bad movement the whole would crumble down, I'm afraid to lose the game!

I see the portrait of a woman of classical beauty, suddenly breaking down into fragments, like in a Picasso's painting.

A pair of glasses I wear shatters in fragments, a motorcycle crumbles in pieces in a parking lot, a cell phone breaks in my hands.

I want to take a taxi but the driver looks very angry, outraged. I get out of the taxi but then realize I've lost my suitcases. I ask two girls I meet in the street for help, they show me the way to the subway but to get there I have to cross a deep forest.

I have to go back to my city, Milan, because of the Covid emergency measures, I take a motorbike but the people in the street seem to look at me in a strange way, I park the motorbike but it falls apart in pieces, I have to find another means of transport now, I am at the parking lot of the train station looking for a taxi, the taxi gets on a train, the train gets on a ferry, I feel as if I were trapped in a series of boxes.

I'm watching a movie about Switzerland, in which 8 soldiers march together with 8 clowns dressed up like birds.

I'm in a square in the mountain, at night, the place could be the arrival of a chairlift, I'm in front of a building with a huge window, it's late at night and very dark, I don't know what I'm doing here and where I could go. I spot in the floor a small window, under it a lighted dining room where an event is going on with many people, they look very happy but they also are too many, I'm scared.

I'm in the Milan Metro at the San Siro station, I realize I've lost my phone and my wallet, I have to go home but I don't know how. I ask a woman for direction and she points me to the close, recently built Three Towers metro station. I look toward the towers and I think that from here the curved one looks more curved than usual.

I am at the seaside, alone, but I can't see the sea, I take a small path and arrive in front of a gigantic EUR-style building (EUR is the name of a Roman borough famous for its impressive architectural style). Inside the building there are no rooms, only niches, each of one is full of people clinging to each other, cheering, there is music and drinks, I don't feel safe there.

A big and beautiful house at dinner time, a party is going on with lot of people but I don't know most of them. I decide to slip away with some friends and we arrive at an amusement park full of oddities, a headless sphinx is playing a concert, people jump in elastic structures, I feel unsafe and want to get out of here quickly.

I'm at home with my partner when a little boy about 10 years old comes in, he's blond, very cute. The person who accompanies him tells me the boy is in foster care and that I should take care of him, but I find out that his father is a murderer, I'm worried because I think I can't trust him.

I'm in a farmhouse with an old small lady, next to us in the floor lies a giant light bulb. An electrician arrives and the old lady asks him to screw in the bulb for light. Will it work?

I ask the electrician, I don't know, he replies, the house is very cold, it will cost a lot to lighten it.

I'm with a friend, we're talking to the Italian politician and former Prime Minister Matteo Renzi, I don't like him, I tell him what I think of him, but he laughs slyly as if he was making fun of me.

The end of the lockdown is just around the corner but the emergency does not seem to be over, and it is overly difficult to imagine what to expect beyond the doorstep. The third Social Dreaming Matrix tells of a distorted world, in which everything is falling in pieces impossible to hold together.

In the dreams, however, the exploration of the what we imagine the new world would be outside has already begun, a journey through an ominous landscape, to an uncertain destination. We get easily lost in our own city whose streets we no longer recognize, everything that once was familiar looks hostile now, when seen from a different angle. Underground stations are hidden by forests of trees; the usual means of transport function in a bizarre way, stuck one into another, a taxi that mounts on top of a train, which in turn gets into a ship.

All along the way we ask for directions to suspicious-looking wayfarers, who show us the way through a forest, up to an underground subway line that will finally take us to destination but in a place that is very different from the one we had in mind. We unintentionally leave our luggage on the ground, drive a scooter that fall in pieces, take a taxi with a scaring taxi driver.

We feel lost in a surreal, distorted, grotesque landscape (see Fig. 3.8), at the mercy of strange characters, an old lady hooks a giant light bulb, we ask for directions to all kind of weird people who can hardly be trusted, we are told that a blond angel-like child could be the son of a murderer. The streets of the city are almost deserted, but the building's basements are full people partying and drinking, unaware of the pandemic.

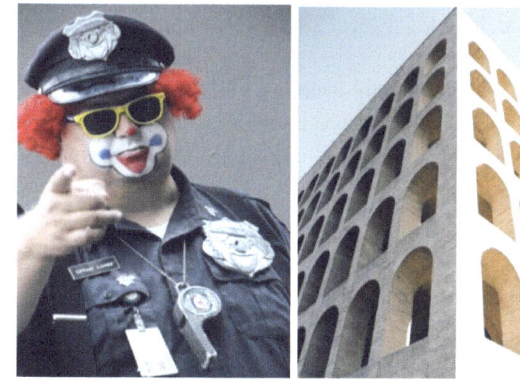
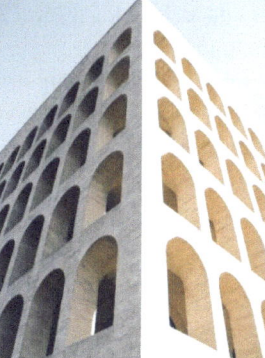
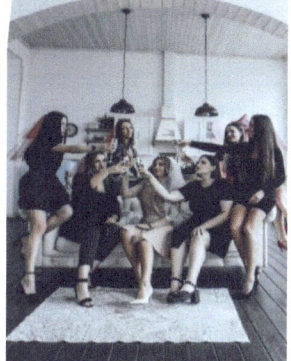

Policemen Clown Dressed
Photo by Steve Harrris on Unsplash

Giant Building
Photo by Andrea Zanenga on Unsplash

People at a Party
Photo by Ann Danilina on Unsplash

Fig. 3.8 Dreams from the imaginary of research, between the grotesque and the journey of discovery

We leave a too crowded party to end up in a creepy amusement park populated by caryatids with cracked faces and huge feet, like images of a Fellini's movie.

It is a world after a tsunami where all the rules have been broken, in which the political power of establishing new rules to manage the pandemic emergency is handled by the controversial Italian political leader Matteo Renzi, heedless of the widespread malaise, who mocks the general bewilderment.

In such a strange landscape we are completely disoriented, always getting lost and confused, our wandering makes no sense. As in a complex puzzle we try to hold together a reality that is falling apart, but the fragments do not fit, we feel lost in a foreign territory.

There is no time to think too much wether the strange characters we meet along the way—the friendly child son of a murderer, the old lady and her strange connection to a bizarre electrician— are trustworthy or not, we have to rely on our instinct and intuition.

Surprisingly enough, the initial discouragement leaves room to a faint tiny hope that the new landscape may give rise to unexpected discoveries.

> A Swiss friend plays electronic music, the sound is like the song of the waves, reminds me of the whale's song.
> I am taking an Excel computer course in an old stone building, the teachers are monks, they all are wearing the monks tunic dress, at the end of the large room there is a door, I tell myself I must go through, behind that door I will find the answers I am looking for.
> I remember a dream I had many years ago, just after the tsunami in Thailand. I was in my office with a former colleague, we waited for the arrival of the tsunami but before leaving we had to arrange some big files, my mother was with us, she was folding my coloured T-shirts, we won't be able to leave on time I thought, we will not be saved.
> I'm looking for the small path which leads to a beach I love very much. I want to show the beach to my granddaughter, but I cannot find the way to get to it anymore.

Animals, that were the main protagonists of the dreams in the first and the second Matrices, seem now to have disappeared from the scene. Only the whale appears, both a mammal and a fish, the largest animal on earth, which is able to inhabit the depths of the sea and can rise to the sky with a flash. The whale symbol of death and rebirth, of introspection and solitude.

The whale is equipped with an evolved brain structure similar to ours, has a sophisticated communication system able to use a very large scale of frequency modulations, unparalleled in the natural world. The song of the whales is at the same time fascinating and dreadful, capable to seduce the sailors and to lead them to disaster.

Like Moby Dick in Melville's famous novel, the whale symbolizes man's perennial struggle on the border between destruction and rebirth.

The whale conjures up the spirit of the abyss, the great Leviathan, a monster of abnormal size. Yet, the whale is believed to be capable of offering salvation and protection in its belly, as happened i.e. to the prophet Jonah in the Bible, and to the puppet Pinocchio in the Carlo Goldoni's novel, who were both rescued from the sea and brought ashore by a whale.

The relationship between the inner and the outer world—represented by the uncanny in the first Matrix, the fragmentation in the second Matrix—takes on now

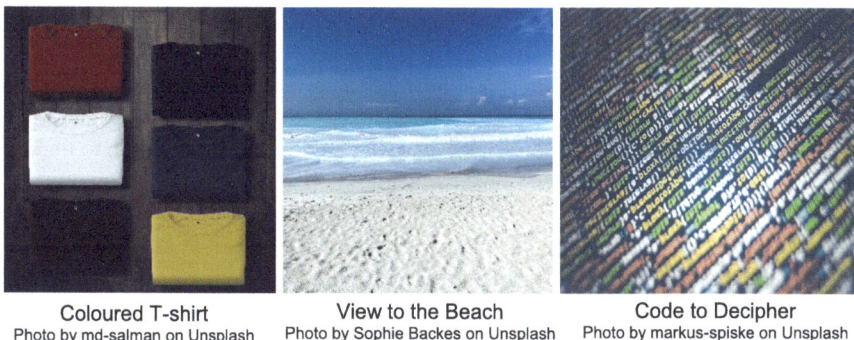

Coloured T-shirt	View to the Beach	Code to Decipher
Photo by md-salman on Unsplash	Photo by Sophie Backes on Unsplash	Photo by markus-spiske on Unsplash

Fig. 3.9 Dreams from the imaginary, between utopia and reality

gigantic, abnormal shapes, and/or infinitely small proportions, which reflect the grotesque surprising transformations of the world we imagine we'll find outside. This world is the world of the Shadow, and the enterprise to accomplish is an introspective journey into the psychic interiority, enduring the bewilderment of potentially frightening discoveries (see Fig. 3.9).

The darkest shadow, and the great unknown mystery, is the relationship with the other, the grotesque characters we encounter along the way. We don't know yet whether they are resources that could guide us with useful advices, dangerous enemies, or just empty appearances, projections of our fears. They may be deceptive presences, like the shadows of the dead that Ulysses encounters on the threshold of Hades on his descent to the underworld, but we still need their guidance.

3.5.3   The Myth Emergent from the Matrix: Ulysse's Descent into the Underworld

Ulysses, the hero par excellence of the "nostos", the return, descended into the underworld before embarking on the journey back to Ithaca to question the clairvoyant Tiresias about the obstacles he would have encountered on his journey.

The descent into the underworld was called in ancient Greece "nekyia", the necromantic ritual of meeting the souls of the dead that symbolizes the process of introversion of the conscious mind venturing into the deepest layers of the unconscious psyche. The nekyia however is not only the fall into the abyss of the deaths, but is also as a significant "catabasis" which allows to meet the archetypal figures populating the unconscious realm. The journey to the underworld is a perilous journey that can bring one to the brink of psychosis; but it is also the way in which the conscious ego can recognise unexpected inner resources of which it was unaware, through which a process of progressive self-expansion becomes possible.

The images of the coffins with the bodies of the virus' victims broadcasted by the media 24/7 during the pandemic emergency sounded like a constant reminder of the existence of the "world of the dead." Even though during the lockdown we tried to forget how close the presence of the underworld was, containing the dead into hospitals and hospices, the underworld resurfaced in the dreams, to remind us that it can no longer be pushed aside, that it is no longer possible to avoid coming to terms with it. However, dreams also tell us that we have already crossed the threshold, that the introspective journey of exploration of the new world has begun, that the creative roots of the unconscious that may live in dreams are essentia, to undertake a new phase of life. Because of the pandemic we had to leave behind an utopian world, the memory of which is comforting and cozy but frozen in time, whose vivid memories have suddenly become simulacra of a past which is now empty of meaning. At the end of the matrix, the images of a dance remind to this inner movement of transformation. They are the images, projected all around the world, of the "dance of the spirits" of the inhabitants of Wuhan, the city in China where the pandemic started, at the reopening of the city; images of a ritual dance that has the enchantment of Japanese Butoh; images of a "glacial tango" that is always danced in pairs. All dances mimicking the irreducible distance that separates life and death in a world deprived of rituals for a collective mourning. If it is a dance of rebirth or a dance of ghosts, is still an open question.

3.5.4 The Habitat of the Third Matrix

From the dream images emerges that the relationship between the outer world and the inner world is played out in two pairs of opposites: Reality versus Utopia and Research Journey versus Grotesque, as we depicted in the third Habitat (see Fig. 3.10).[4] The images in Fig. 3.10 are part of the imaginary dreamed and evoke the two pairs of opposites.

Opposition Between Utopia and Reality In dreams we set out on a journey and start wandering around in cities where it is easy to get lost, whose streets we no longer recognize, where everything that was familiar seems now to be weird. The journey is a quest and at the same time a journey into the unknown, like Ulysses' return to Ithaca, marked by the song of the whales that captivates the sailors. But the journey is also Switzerland, a destination that alludes to an orderly and peaceful world that nevertheless conceals many oddities, in which Utopia and Reality are mixed up.

Opposition Between Journey of Research and Grotesque The world we discover outside is deformed, fragmented, a scattered reality which is difficult to hold together. The wonderful coincides with the terrible, "the others" have the disturbing features of the shadow. In this world, however, humans return to prominence, with alternating emotions ranging from fear to hope, from surprise to aggression.

---

[4]Photos by Mark Basarab (Reality), Gabriel Dizzi (Utopia), Andy Beales (Research Journey), Alice (Grotesque) on Unsplash.

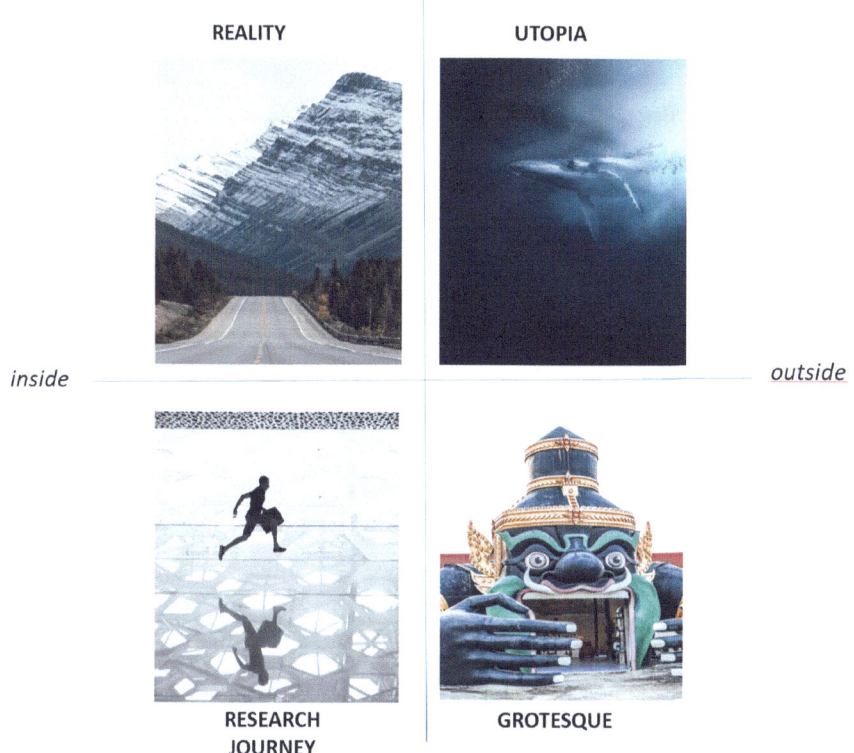

Fig. 3.10 Habitat of April 15th 2020

3.5.4.1   Key Points of the Third Matrix

- Utopia and Reality: The old world has fallen in pieces, but the desire for rebirth is still an unattainable utopia.
- Research Journey and Grotesque: the Journey brings to light a distorted reality, the projection of our fears, where the wondrous coincides with the awful.
- The "helpers" figures found along the way represent the arising of hope.
- Surprise, improvisation, playfulness are resources for a renewal.

Key emerging question:
Are the helpers trustworthy? Or are they only
shadows of our fears?

3.6   Fourth Social Dreaming Matrix: 5th of May 2020 Revelation, Discovery, Return

3.6.1   The Socio-Political Context at the Time

The end of the lockdown was officially due on May 4th 2020, but we were far from the return to a normal life. The curve of the virus had not significantly decreased and the Prime Minister Giuseppe Conte, in his long-awaited discourse that should have sanctioned the end of the lockdown, made it clear that we were still far from the end of the emergency, and consequently most of the restrictions should remain in place.

In fact, few amendments to the most binding rules were done at the reopening: traveling within the country was allowed only to visit family members and relatives, which ensued endless discussions about who were the relatives, if friends, acquaintances, boyfriends/girlfriends, lovers were included in the category. Most of the shops remained closed with rare exceptions like hairdressers and beauty parlors, but the reasons behind those exceptions were not clear. Bars and restaurants were allowed to work only on take-away service: Walking in streets and parks, practicing outdoor activities, was permitted only at a safe distance, carefully established by law. Any kind of gatherings inside and outside the house were strictly forbidden, and even the number of the diners that could be hosted at home was set to a maximum of six people.

The government stated they were planning an exit from the emergency "with caution," which became the new mantra of the summer. Meanwhile, a large array of ubiquitous video-virologists debated in the media everything and its opposite, highly contributing to increase the general confusion. The result was a huge bewilderment, the most restrictive rules that were seriously affecting the lives of people remaining in place. Schools and companies could only work on remote, which officially opened endless discussions about the pros and cons of "smart working" and "distance learning," issues which are still under public debate.

All these explosive contradictions, however, reinforced the idea that the virus was not the cause, but the accelerator of a process of fragmentation of the social context and the rules that hold people together, which was already at work under the surface before the pandemic. The spread of the virus has made these contradictions more visible and palpable, shedding light on uncomfortable issues.

Will we be able in the future to manage the fractures that undermine our society in the long term, not only in the face of an emergency? Will we be able to set up long-term projects for the inclusion of the weak, the fragile, the marginalized, instead of imposing constraints that imply prohibitions and punishments and limit the freedom of all?

3.6.2   The Inner World at May 5: Images from the Dreams

I'm flying high in the sky, with open hands, in the midst of floating colored scarves.
A beautiful young girl, dressed in colors, she is pregnant, full of life, I'm staring at her in amazement.
A duck with a bright yellow beak suddenly emerges from a burrow on the bank of a pond.

I'm walking barefoot in a lake of jelly-like fluid, green, candy-colored water, the feeling is warm and pleasant, it's a wonderful sensation. Along with me many people, among them I spot Madonna (the singer), she greets me, we walk together in the water.

I'm growing a fragrant rose on the balcony of my house, I love this flower, when I realize that someone has stolen it, I'm desperate.

I'm staring in amazement the magnificent view of a lake from the window of my house terrace, feeling a profound sense of peace.

I walk knee-deep in a blue lagoon, the water is wonderful, clear and crystalline, suddenly a huge wave rises up and drags me to the bottom of the sea, I'm not scared though, I realize I can swim and breathe underwater like a fish, around me many colorful beautiful fishes.

I am sitting on a large green meadow stroking the soft coat of a lamb, it's a beautiful moment of peace, suddenly I find a zip on the lamb's coat, I unzip it and realize there's only a skeleton under the mantle.

I run along the Serio riverbed in a foggy evening, silence around, suddenly black huge parallelepipeds start falling from the sky, a gigantic typhoon sweeps away the landscape, a large tower crashes, I see boys falling to the ground at my feet, the typhoon has red-orange eyes like a big squid.

I see a black moon, like an eclipse, in front of the moon the shadow of the earth.

The dreams of the fourth Social Dreaming Matrix on May 5th 2020, at the end of the 2 months of lockdown, celebrate the rediscovery of sensoriality through the vitality of all the senses, from sight to touch, from taste to smell. A carousel of vivid, strong, colorful sensations enshrines the promise of pleasure and rebirth, and the nature looses the threatening aspects that had so much space in the previous matrices and returns to be a source of well-being, joy, and life.

In the dreams we are keen to rediscover pleasurable sensations, immersed in a vital nature that enables us to fly in the sky and to breathe underwater like fishes.

Surprisingly, the fear has disappeared and we can easily adapt to the new world of crystal-clear waters, blue deep-green lakes, flowered meadows under boundless skies. Images of pregnant, smiling women are dressed in bright colors (see Fig. 3.11). In the dreams we rediscover a long-forgotten well-being that sounds like the promise of an intense pleasure and the expectation of a renewal.

Beautiful images follow one another like in a film sequence, along the way we meet movie stars like Madonna, Al Pacino, and Joe Pesci, fantastic literary characters like Harry Potter, we see the towers of Hogwarts and the Little Prince's rose.

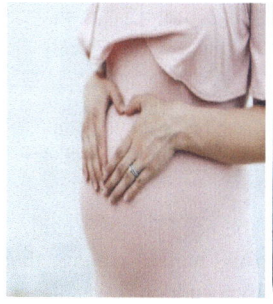 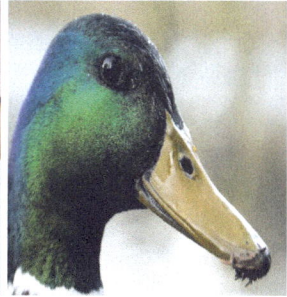 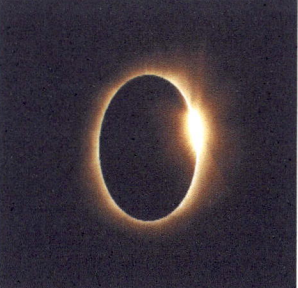

Pregnant woman
Photo by Juan Encalada on Unsplash

Duck with a big yellow beak
Photo by Kris Mikael Krister on Unsplash

Moon Ecplipse
Photo by Jongsun Lee on Unsplash

Fig. 3.11 Dreams from the imaginary, between hyperreality and hallucination

As in a game of mirrors, the rediscovery of the senses refers to the search for meaning, in a game of altered significance in which, as someone pointed out, it seems that the unconscious had a lot of fun muddying the waters.

However, the hyperreality enhanced by the sensorial experience is ultimately intoxicating. Gradually we discover, in fact, that the seemingly, beautiful augmented reality might actually contain the hope of a new life, embodied by pregnant women and initiation rituals, such as walking in shallow waters. But suddenly, just when we feel we are finally ready to happily embrace the new world, something horrible happens. The little lamb we were peacefully caressing turns out to be a skeleton, a black moon appears in the sky covering the view of the earth, a gigantic orange squid sweeps over us like a cyclone. The expectation of long-awaited change is so high, we seek a rebirth, we long for the empowerment of energies and resources, we dream of soaring through the air with open arms and breathing underwater.

But the sudden switch from Hyperreality to Hallucination discloses the two opposites poles of reality.

Hyperreality has the vital charge of sensuality and pleasure, profound sensations that we have been deprived of for so long and missed so much.

Hallucination, however, opens up a different dimension that is inaccessible without an altered state, an intermediate dimension that lies between the sensible and the intelligible worlds. A dimension that conceals, superpowers we are unable to master, behind which lurks the danger of an ego inflation.

> I am on the set of a movie with all the crew, we are waiting for the arrival of the director Maresco to start filming. While we wait we pass around an album of old photos, they are out of focus and confused, the time goes and the director does not show up, his chair remains empty.
>
> I'm putting order to a drawer full of old recipes, I try to figure out a method to sort them, the image is clear as if in a movie, I think I need to find an organizing principle to fix things up.
>
> I'm in an underground warehouse, the walls around me are shrinking, I'm in danger but manage to get out of it. Outside a car is waiting for me with two mafia bosses inside, they are the movie stars Al Pacino and Joe Pesci, I think they want to kill me and punch them in the face, they fall down, then get up and congratulate me, they tell me I'm a brave good fellow.
>
> I am at the University of Mathematics in Dusseldorf, the huge building looks like the Harry Potter's college of Hogwarts, the sky is dark, inside the building there are dormitories with many children. The teachers invite me to a party in a circus tent, I get inside the tent and sit close to a woman, two students and a 8 years old boys, we are sitting on a sauna-like bench when some air starts to come out from small holes under the bench, I know I'm breathing hallucinogenic substances, I fear I'm addicted, I realize I'm in danger, suddenly I realize the circus hides an abuse of children.
>
> I am in a beauty shop, the saleswoman is pregnant, she is nice and talkative, but I'm struck by her gaze, she has blue eyes but one of them is open and the other is stitched shut. She holds a magazine and wants to show me an article about her daughter, the article is of hers future success.

The creative flair of the sensorial experience counterpoints the need for an organizing principle, a method to "put order in the drawers" that could help to manage the new situation, avoiding the risk of being taken by surprise by a sudden reversal.

Dealing with movie stars and fairy tale characters who take turns in such bizarre ways is not easy: at first glance the two "mafiosi" Al Pacino and Joe Pesci look

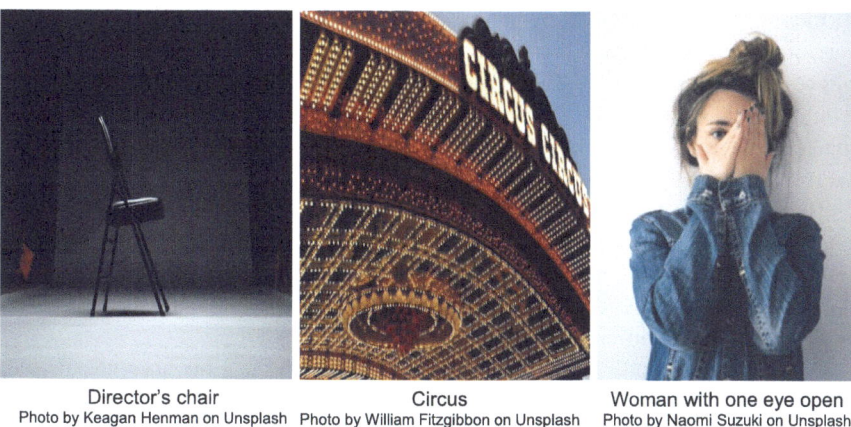

Director's chair	Circus	Woman with one eye open
Photo by Keagan Henman on Unsplash	Photo by William Fitzgibbon on Unsplash	Photo by Naomi Suzuki on Unsplash

Fig. 3.12 Imaginary from the Fourth Matrix, between creativity and hypercontrol

menacing, with a gun in their fists, but in the end they turn out to be cheering old friends. A beautifully impressive giant squid hovers in an orange post-atomic sky. I walk with Madonna in a pool of green jelly, I breed a rose like that of the Little Prince. However, there is no order to the sequence of the images, there is no director to lead the game; and while we wait for him, his chair remains empty and everything gets confused (see Fig. 3.12).

The newborn creativity is evoked in the dreams by images of pregnant women glowing with life. The creative flair is entirely feminine, generative, powerful, magical, inspires hope and respect. The image of the feminine evoked by the dreams is not, however, the overwhelming image of the Great Mother emboding the power of Nature.

The image of the feminine is a pregnant woman who looks toward the future, an image of "Anima" with the gift of prophecy represented by a woman with one eye open and the other stitched shut, inviting to reconcile the outer gaze with an inner vision that brings wisdom and vision (see Fig. 3.12). A woman with the gift of prophecy like Cassandra the unfortunate princess of Troy, a gift which is both a power and a curse.

3.6.3   The Myth Emergent from the Matrix: Cassandra the Unfortunate Prophetess

Cassandra, daughter of Priam, princess of Troy and priestess of Apollo, had received the gift of prophecy from the god as a pledge of his love. But after her refusal to give herself to him, Apollo turned the gift he had made into a curse. Cassandra could indeed see the future, but no one would believe her prophecies of doom. She knew in advance of Troy's destruction, she knew the fate the gods had in store for her loved ones and for herself; but no one believed her warnings, and her prophecies of doom condemned her to isolation and to living in anticipation of the misfortunes she knew she could not avoid.

At the end of the matrix, Hypercontrol and Creativity, symbolizing the dominant masculine and the generative feminine, remain two irretrievably separate worlds whose composition is impossible. The profound longing for a new world richer in "soul" is held back by the sterile wait for a director, expected to bring order in chaos. And the inward-looking eye of prophecy is rendered blind and impotent by the ruthless need for control of a vigilant conscience that will not let go.

The opposition between Creativity and Hypercontrol performs the eternal challenge between Dionysus and Apollo, the Dionysian world of the sensorial elation colliding with the Apollonian rationality of the control upon reality.

The Apollonian, hyperactive, one-sided, masculine strategy has proved to be ineffective to find a different way to relate with nature.

Dionysus, it is worth to mention, was the god of women, his ancient cult was predominantly sacred to women. The female images of pregnant women of the dreams had an unattainable beauty, but their voice remained ultimately unheard, confined in the madness of hallucinations.

Like in a Dyonisian rite, the images of the feminine suggest the possibility of a transformation, hoping for a reunion that could ultimately happen. But, like in a Dyonisian rite, they are still crushed by the fears of losing the rational hypercontrol and the long-awaited pregnancies turn out to be, at the end, hysterical pregnancies.

3.6.4 The Habitat of the Fourth Matrix

From the dream images, it emerges that the relationship between the outer and the inner world is played out in two pairs of opposites: Creativity versus Hypercontrol and Hallucination versus Hyperreality, as we depicted in the fourth Habitat (see Fig. 3.13). Images in Fig. 3.13[5] are part of the imaginary dreamed and evoke the two pairs of opposites.

Opposition Between Hyperreality and Hallucination The rediscovery of sensoriality through the reawakening of the senses, from sight to touch, from taste to smell, gives rise to vivid, strong, vital sensations, promises of rebirth. The nature loses the disturbing and threatening aspects that had so much space in the previous matrices and becomes a source of well-being and joy, a new source of life. However, disturbing and hallucinatory aspects suddenly emerge, and the beautiful expectation of a rediscovered Eden turns into a nightmare.

Opposition Between Creativity and Hypercontrol The creativity evoked by the images of pregnant women is totally feminine, potentially generative. The image of

---

[5]Photos by Charles Eugene (Creativity), Jan Antonin Kolar (Hypercontrol), Joshua Fuller (Hallucination), Alex Gruber (Hyperreality) on Unsplash.

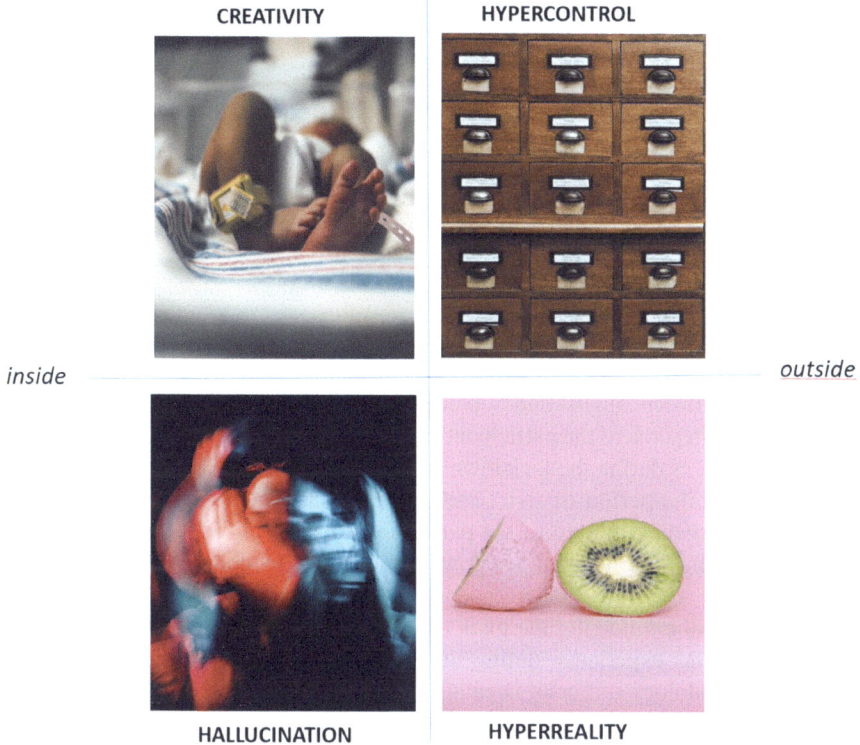

Fig. 3.13 The habitat of May 5th 2020

the feminine is powerful, magical, prophetic, symbolizes the invisible and the transcendent, looks toward the future. However, the female creativity is blocked by the need for a vigilant hypercontrolling conscience that does not let go of its grip on reality. The need for hypercontrol hides the fear of losing control, of being overwhelmed by the senses, in a strange game of altering meanings in which it seems that the unconscious has had a lot of fun muddling the waters.

3.6.5 Key Points of the Fourth Matrix

- Hyperreality and Hallucination: we rediscover the pleasure of the senses, and the nature as source of pleasure. But is this all real?
- Creativity and Hypercontrol: The generative power of the feminine (prophecy) is blocked by a defensive consciousness.
- The visible and the invisible, which one should we rely on? What hides behind the appearances of a new reality?

Key emerging question:

Are the new pregnancies a promise of rebirth or

are they only hysterical pregnancies?

3.7   Feedback from the Participants

In the period between August and September 2021, we conducted a small qualitative research with some of the participants involved in the experience of the 4 Social Dreaming matrices during the lockdown in Italy (March–May 2020).

At that time the period of strict lockdown in Italy had passed, even though the health emergency related to the pandemic was still an issue monitored and controlled at the institutional level with measures to contain the spread of contagions.

We report in the following the main evidence from the interviews with participants of the SDM experience during the pandemic with some useful reflections about the methodology of Social Dreaming.

A total of 6 one-hour telephone interviews were conducted. The interviewees were "dreamers" who had taken part in one or more matrices, enrolled on a voluntary basis. The interviews were recorded with people's consent and analyzed anonymously with respect to privacy.

The research carried out was aimed at retrieving the experience in order to acquire useful information for systematizing the SD method and analyzing, after time, the benefits and possible applications in the post-pandemic context.

Interviews were based on a semi-structured guideline that touched on these points:

- The Social Dreaming experience during lockdown.

  - Meaning for oneself.
  - Relevant aspects of the experience.
  - Learnings from the experience.
  - Evaluation of the online mode.

- Role of the SD methodology in the future.

Below are presented the results collected, aggregated around the research questions we made.

- What did the Social Dreaming experience during lockdown represent to you at that time?
- What were the most relevant aspects of the experience?

- What did you learn on a more strictly personal level?
- The online mode was a constraint, but at the same time a challenge. How was your experience of the online matrix?
- Thinking about the days ahead, the context has changed but we still remain in a situation conditioned by the pandemic, could Social Dreaming play a role in this context? Which one?
- Could this be a useful tool to repurpose? Why? With what purpose?
- What mode would be desirable?
- What value might it have? For whom especially?

These following pages outline the results of this follow-up, question by question.

"What did the Social Dreaming Experience during lockdown represent to you at that time?"

The SDM experience was for many of the participants one of the first initiatives aimed to collectively process the pandemic applying psychodynamic tools. Most of them experienced it in a positive way, as a very helpful necessary experience at this moment, characterized by closure, isolation, strong feelings of fears and anxiety.

> One of the first collective initiatives with psychodynamic methods to collectively process the pandemic, a space to reprocess that traumatic experience. I remember Social Dreaming and another pathway initiated by Coirag almost at the same time through the Operational Group tool.
> It was like a gift… It was crucial, I think I looked for you… I felt like I didn't have time and space, energy, power to do anything.

The space of Social Dreaming was described as an open space, in which was possible "to let things go," refresh oneself, recover some energy and the contact with other people experiencing similar situation that the lockdown had taken away.

The dream exchange was a time that allowed "getting lost" while at the same time staying grounded to something tangible, the collective dimension opening up to the capacity of self-reflection.

> In that moment it was a clearing, an unfilled empty space where I could imagine, let go, be in a group, feel less alone, where I could have more power than the helpless and saturated state of the first lockdown….
> A window, a contact, a connection with other people very useful and necessary to keep in touch with other people, but not only that… also a moment of deep reflection…

Engaging with others was of great help to break the feelings of solitude, but the group dimension seemed nonetheless to be missing. Rather than on interaction, the group dynamic worked on an affective level, though still anchored to a collective dimension. Relationships with others were described as weak, but only marginally experienced as lacking. The interviewed reported that "we were all in the same situation," they did not feeling alone.

The image that emerged was of many individualities doing "something for themselves" (finding comfort, well-being, relief, etc.) rather than a group engaged in a task (some underlined the difference from other experiences lived at that same time, based on other group methodologies as in example Operational Group, where instead there was interaction and mutual recognition).

> Discovering that others had dreams similar to yours....
>
> It was a time to compare and exchange experiences with others… a time also to reflect on how it was going on a personal level.
>
> My relational memory was of struggling to perceive the group, being in the group, there were so many individualities… there was a feeling that we were not a group. We made the effort to position ourselves on dreams….
>
> A time of comfort, we were all experiencing the same situation. Having the same world-view, fears, hearing that emotions were felt by others helped to make sense

Social Dreaming certainly stimulated the exploration of the unknown: being part of a group with no specific goal, feeling contained in a secure safe space, sharing ones dreams with barely known people, was an experience of lightening from the heaviness of the days and of freedom of the mind, of wandering around with no limits. An empty space that at that moment acted as a counterbalance to the high tension of being overwhelmed by the daily news.

> Navigating anxieties and fears together with others, becoming aware of a number of elements, it was a bit of walking into the unknown.
>
> Metaphorical, imaginative tool, let the mind wander… it was a space to vent without venting.
>
> A space for reflection and escapism… There was anxiety and anguish about what was happening, you couldn't get out

"What were the most relevant aspects of the experience?"

The deconstruction of the setting amplified the dimension of exploration, abandonment, discovery of common themes brought in by multiple dreams that seemed to form a collective plot.

The setting fostered the entry into a sleep-like state of mind, thus creating a very powerful sense of trust of being in a secure space.

> The first meeting, it was the discovery of a situation where I don't know where it's going to go or where it's going to take us, but it seems like a situation that can do me good…
>
> Seeing how after the first meetings themes emerged, the possibility of making hypotheses about themes that were obviously affecting the collective… the relationship with nature, what with the reporting and the video made it evident… Seeing how out of these very unstructured situations came very pragmatic possibilities, making hypotheses about what is happening to the collective, to the subject in an intersubjective situation
>
> The impression of going into an altered state of consciousness, a kind of dormancy, an expanded mental state between wakefulness and sleep, with a slight loss of the boundary of the self

Some themes stuck out the most, especially Nature erasing the spaces of Culture. It struck the pragmatic aspect of the methodology, which, while starting from an unstructured setting, was able to identify themes for reflection that led to questioning and reflecting in a very concrete way on what was happening in the collective dimension.

> Dreams about nature, of an uninhabited world with nature taking over. Feeling a little less in control of the world….

> Speaking of the plants, a trifle -- I had changed the arrangement of plants in the furniture.

Also relevant was the experience of the lack of the group dimension (a disappointment for someone), which nevertheless reinforced the intention of a methodology that seemed aimed at connecting individuals within a larger collective dimension rather than with each other.

> Vague group, there was no eye contact or relational
>
> There was the possibility of oscillating from an individual dimension to opening up to a long-term story, e.g., the relationship with illness, with death, animals, the recovery of bestiality in natural spaces… it was generative, my attention shifted to these cues, it was an opportunity to elaborate, an anticipation on the level of the image of what emerged later on the rational level… like seeds bearing fruit…
>
> The experience really struck me, the commonalities and dissonances of dreams between people, as if there is a colloid that unites us
>
> I had participated to other Social Dreaming in-person experiences, there was also a sense of estrangement, but looking at each other in person allowed for interaction. The whole online experience was more between strangers, there was no mutual recognition. This thing I missed…
>
> It wasn't group. It's you with the monitor. There is no we, everyone is on their own. There is no eye contact, there is a lack of closeness.

"What did you learn on a more strictly personal level?"

Learning from experience was described in personal terms:

- Personal well-being
- A key insight into ongoing change
- Increased self-awareness exploration of inner space
- Acceptance of the unknown
- Recognizing oneself in collective archetypes
- Dream fragments, even in the long run: Transgenerational, archaic images of connection between the individual dimension and openness to the collective.

It is especially the first part of the dream exchange that was credited with bringing to consciousness and verbalizing contents of self and recognizing oneself in a collective archetypal dimension.

> A tool that helps to have greater awareness, the meetings were useful for reflection.
>
> I realized how valuable the first phase is, soaking in the collective unconscious… a more expressive, associative, phrase of loss and daze…. and how much instead the interpretation, activation of the cognitive part risks bringing the whole thing down to something known, less special, less unique and useful…
>
> SD is a tool that helped you become aware and verbalize. I became aware that I was going through an experience of danger, never experienced before, of disrupting my life-styles. The fear, the overwhelm that the virus brought, the idea of loss and death. I became aware that life does not run on established tracks….
>
> Discovering that others had dreams similar to yours….
>
> The lockdown space represented the possibility to separate from the social space and recover, explore the inner space. It also had a long-term effect. Transgenerational images--for example, the plague of the 600s.

It was a kind of processing, becoming aware, especially recognizing oneself in a humanity, collective archetypes… it helped me to become aware and verbalize from the dreams, give form to the contents that came…

The thing I took home with me? The reconfirmation of this collective dimension of humanity, archetypes that give meaning to the experience you are having, being able to not be overwhelmed by events…

It's a great way to look inside a little bit, to compare myself with others, to have a different point with which to look at reality, especially at that time when there was no possibility of feeling free to express yourself…

In addition to the individual benefits, some also emphasized the methodological aspects as an important acquisition. First and foremost, the discovery of a method that allowed people to listen to each other and express otherwise unspeakable experiences, thanks to the capacity of the setting to create an intimate atmosphere between people who were also, in part, strangers to each other, but always in a "lay" way, without the implications of psychotherapy.

A way to talk about uncomfortable things in a group in a secular way, without psychotherapy….

Personal well-being, related to sharing with others, not feeling alone … the other benefit was having a key to interpret reality. For example, the theme of the fall of civilization and severe natural events destroying civilization…

The host's approach of asking questions and making assumptions rather than giving interpretations and answers was also considered facilitating.

How different it is to hypothesize versus to interpret, they are two modes…I was already coming from a school that pushes me to hypothesize and less to interpret and there I had confirmation that cognitively using the material that experience brings out to make hypotheses, which are more light, open, precarious than instead of using what emerges from experience to go and confirm that one a thought that I already have but this is less generative…in SD there are both possibilities to be able to go through…

Hypothesizations can open up multiple readings and at a time like this of discontinuity I find it more useful to ask questions and hypotheses and based on that activate actions…

The discovery that there is a method, a case for listening to even intimate things… I talked about the dreamed dead in plastic bags, half alive and half dead… a place to express even horrible things that are there and that are part of being human

Hosting was key, sticking to the rules, synthesis work… we tried to make full use of this crop of ideas

The use of "maps" for each matrix was considered useful and intriguing in this regard. Those who recognized the maps as valuable tools were also the most interested on Social Dreaming as a tool for the understanding of the context.

Bateson said the map is the territory, there is no objective territory, work on the maps you have, going in search of maps, seemed to me a very intriguing activity….

More experiencing than understanding

More marginally, especially for those who brought "very strong" materials there was the struggle to remember the experience.

With respect to content, I remember some dreams very well, but today I have a hard time remembering anything that stuck with me, it's as if there was an overall removal of things … the material was strong, perhaps because of this

"The online mode was a constraint, but it was also a challenge. How did you experience the online matrix?"

The online mode, that was initially thought to be a critical element for the establishment of the setting, actually turned out to be the elective dimension for bringing out the collective matrix, connoting the online SD as a distinctive experience compared to the in-presence version (which some participants already had experience of).

The subtraction of the "third dimension," in short, was beneficial in amplifying the elements of setting rarefaction and depersonalization that aided the activity of dream emergence and sharing.

The virtual facilitated the experience of immersion in the collective matrix, strengthening the exploration in the "dark." The prevalence of the virtual dimension over the personal dimension reinforced the sense of rarefaction and is in line with the dreamlike dimension of dreams, imaginative, giving rise to a collective experience (the collective dream) but through a participation that remained strictly individual. It recalled the experience of enjoying a movie at the cinema.

The presence of a depersonalization setting, the slow pace enabled a greater focus on self to be activated in order to go back to the dreams.

Facilitating factors related to the online mode were:

- the virtual dimension (in comparison with the in-presence mode),
- not seeing people, being able to take the video off, disappearance of faces from the screen/camcorder off, not looking into each other's eyes, non-proximity,
- auditory-only contact, background noise, vibration in the background,
- connection from many different cities/many people,
- presence of empty moments,
- still image of the screen,
- slow pace.

In addition to this, the hosting function played a great role in facilitating by

- an approach to hypothesizing rather than interpreting, remaining as open as possible,
- the welcoming ability to accommodate raw materials that have no form, creating a welcoming environment.

A key aspect of managing these meetings was thus to avoid an interpretive approach that would add speed to the SD pace and close down the reflection and thought process around known theses/ideas/patterns.

Virtual might be the elective place for immersion in a collective matrix, some things to me facilitated the immersion…the fact of not seeing people, being able to take the video off…you may leave the microphone on and you feel the vibration in the background…to me the thought of being an astronaut in the cosmos made me feel like an explorer inside a big dark, hooked through…. An explorer floating inside a big dark to explore with this background noise of the open microphones… the possibility then i connect from many places, in many people… I see the merits more than the disadvantages…

The dream basically is approached to the theme of the screen, going to the cinema is a daydream… in that huge screen I experience a state of immersion that I experienced in the SD.

The online nature of SD is an advantage. While in other forms of group discussion presence is enriching, here the virtual, non-personal dimension I found it effective. It is a dreamlike dimension, it reinforces this rarefaction, you are within a group but you are alone, it is almost a collective dream. It facilitated, there were gaps, fixed image, the disappearance of faces from the screen allows you to focus on yourself. Also the pace, it was slow, almost never was it excited talking, a pace that facilitated the connection…

At first I thought the online limited a lot, the turning off the camera, just having the auditory contact, but then…

Online emphasizes the absence of the group even more and thus removes inhibitory brakes, because in presence you have them…

"Thinking about the days ahed, the context has changed, but we still remain in a situation conditioned by the pandemic, could Social Dreaming play a role in this context? Which one?"

Certainly the context was changed from the big wave (tsunami) to the long wave. However, we were still within the pandemic and processes of change, there was a lessening of emotional intensity, albeit with an awareness of lingering malaise.

Suggestions were that SD might have a role as a useful tool in a context of change to intercept how much the situation, collectively, can play a potentially traumatizing role and generate malaise, stress, etc. at the individual level.

We are fully inside, not quite inside the big T, the big trauma…. Maybe for many people and organizations it has become a small T, one of those chronic, minor traumas that you deal with on a daily basis, maybe you forget about but it produces malaise, anxiety, stress… certainly around me I register more anxiety and malaise, less energy than in the pre-covid period.

Now there is a long wave of malaise that is in danger of not being seen by the radar and is in danger, if we don't deal with it, of having really heavy effects in the near future. So for me there is an extreme need for methodologies like SD to try to access radar on what I feel is very active around us in terms of traumatic and potentially traumatizing

"Could this be a useful tool to repurpose? Why? With what purpose?"

Social Dreaming as a tool for analyzing and understanding what is happening at the collective level was certainly considered useful: interviewees used the metaphors of radar, thermometer, deep listening recurs.

It is not a tool that works on the group. An important aspect to keep in mind is how to communicate SD to a potential interlocutor. Communication and compliance may be critical if one nurtures expectations of linear understanding.

I find it less useful as a self standing experience but potentially very useful hooked into intervention projects, where what emerged even or just through SD is used to try to make things happen that go to work on those issues

Is a tool for understanding, but does not allow you to take action

Collective self-analysis tool committed to bringing about change in one's life. It lacks a moment where you plan … projecting into the future, a creative group where people commit to identifying deliverables

Today the situation is a little different, I experience more freedom than I did in the first lockdown, I feel less of a need to compare myself with others… certainly it would make sense but less frequently.

I don't know, maybe to see how people are moving emotionally and collectively. Today it might be useful to see how people are reacting to the pandemic. It might be as useful as taking the temperature.

It's a space of emergence of patterns and thoughts rather than processing them.

I have in mind the comparison with the other experience (reference to the Operations Group), there I have in mind the people, the group, recognition experience. In Social Dreaming the relationship-related dimension disappears.

"What mode would be desirable?"

One area to be developed, they suggested, is Social Dreaming capacity to support processes of change, both for individuals and groups. In this sense, it would be possible to use the tool in an articulated process with other different methodologies. While SD in fact allows for the emergence of recurring themes, it is also true that it does not offer, in its structure, a moment to activate furthermore structured reflections, which at some point would be much needed.

Some interviewees already cited some experiences done by themselves using SD in conjunction with experiential workshops, operational groups, development activities.

We used experiential workshops, we happened to do this for managers, we had them work 4 days in experiential workshops that aimed at institutional transformation and we used daily SD moments, placed at the beginning of the day. They were moments that inhaled, created connection between people, this facilitated the work that was done in the rest of the day, but mostly we as staff used what came from the matrix to make assumptions about the system and to imagine how we could intervene in the laboratory system to try to disrupt it, to push it in some direction that they thought was useful…

It raises an issue of understandability for people not in the field … and then compliance and how much these people rely on the method, instead we risk being closed and buttoned up rather than diving into the matrix.

It could be very useful in organizational development projects at that stage of listening, when you start doing focus groups and interviews to understand how it is…we use at this stage not only the head but we try to get the joys, the rages expressed…why not also be able to add a SD pathway that goes to intercept a collective and deeper dimension

Either you do it every time there is a change of pace, for example in September/October… or it has a recurring pattern over a period of time, six months or a year, where knowledge becomes a theme…

SD could play a role today, but would need to be better understood. Important to define the nature of the participants and the regular cadence.

I would like to do it in a beautiful environment surrounded by nature, there is a need to get back in touch with nature…the location is important, it must be an environment that is familiar with the dream…

In our experience the SD led to the development of ideas, we grounded them… each of us on a stimulus that came from there will give a talk… it was a fertile experience, a diagnostic tool of potential…

"What value might it have? For whom especially?"

The value mostly recognized to Social Dreaming is the function of exploration and anticipation, which is possible because of the SD setting: a place that facilitates the emergence of a dream imagery, the possibility of relying on insights that may also have practical repercussions.

The reprocessing and the interpretation of patterns seem to play a secondary role, and their pursuit may represent a risky zone. The expectation of using SD with the claim of understanding what is going on by making too many interpretations could lead to strong disappointments.

> It is a need for analysis that sociologists, psychologists, those who deal with the human have at times of discontinuity, when there is a need to understand what is going on, what time has ended and what times might begin… and at this stage of analysis I am always more convinced by those who work by the path of hypotheses than those who follow more clear-cut paths, linked to an interpretive process…
>
> You have to engage those who want to understand. What do ordinary people dream about? The real problem is to give elements to recompose society. In the last SD I felt a refined elite, of old gentlemen reflecting…
>
> In general one would need to find a target audience interested in understanding, a less rationalized approach…. Those who as a result of the pandemic feel that things should not go back to the way they were before
>
> A lot of value on developing and diagnosing the real problems…

Some areas of intervention are considered elective because they have been more impacted by the long wave of the pandemic. Certain roles, more than others, manifest high stress signals related to the challenges they had faced since the beginning of the pandemic, to which they are still exposed because of the uncertain scenario. More generally, SD was considered a useful tool for those who experience change with tension and difficulties within organizations.

Eventually, SD is a tool for the understanding of the most hidden layers of reality; works as an emotional glue, but, most of all, is an educational tool to develop those qualities that are today more useful as ever in scenarios of turbulent change: the capacity to surrender/to abandon the paradigm of control/the capacity to leave to uncertain destinations/a self-reflective attitude.

> It is the age that requires the courage not of recklessness, but of aimless departure….
>
> SD could also be educational for skills that are needed at this moment in history… in part it is needed to surrender, to let go, to not seek certainty and control…but it is the time to gain the capacity for surrender, against the performance society that always wants you to be on the piece and never give up…where you accept losing control, latching on to something or others you don't yet have full knowledge or trust of… the ability to dare, to do new things, the ability to challenge your prejudices, the courage to take risks…courage also to immerse yourself in the matrix, to make a fool of yourself to step out of the image of the woman/man who always has all the answers…great flexibility
>
> It's also a method of educating in those very useful skills for better living at a time in history like this….
>
> One possible avenue is to hook SD into tools that work on group or individual counseling pathways.

Mentioned as possible elective targets: medical/health care personnel, school personnel, managers, and business leaders.

Certainly all the populations under attack, all the health care sector, even all the positions of responsibility in companies… the issue of being a leader in today's world of work, being responsible for people, there's exhorbitant pressure… so many people are jumping in, they're going out… the teaching field, faculty … partly because there is little energy or desire to make the triple pike jump that the historical moment requires and partly because there are so many people leaving to retrieve old degrees to join the school lists…

A tool that gives an interpretive key to action, useful for people who have people management responsibilities

It would serve to understand how much we are getting used to this life, stay in touch with the disease that continues to be there, useful especially for the most impacted categories, e.g. school.

References

1. Barthes R. Introduction to the structural analysis of narratives. In: Encyclopedia of semiotics. London: Oxford University Press; 1966.
2. Field S. The Screenwriter's workbook. New York: Dell Publishing Co.; 1984.
3. Corbetta P. La ricerca sociale: metodologia e tecniche, vol. III. Milano: Le tecniche qualitative/Il Mulino; 2015b.
4. Corbetta P. La ricerca sociale: metodologia e tecniche, vol. I. Milano: I paradigmi di riferimento/Il Mulino; 2015a.
5. Riessman CK. Narrative analysis. London: Sage; 1993.
6. Atkinsons RG. The life story interview (qualitative research methods). London: Sage; 1998.
7. Gabriel Y. The uses of stories. In: The life story interview (qualitative research methods). London: Sage; 1998. p. 135–60.
8. Hillman J. Saggio su Pan. Milano: Adelphi; 2013.

Chapter 4
Dreams, Symbols, Narratives: Dream as a Space of Imagination

4.1 The Social Function of Dreams

> This mood makes itself felt everywhere, politically, socially and philosophically. "We are living in what the Greeks called the Kairos - the right time - for a metamorphosis of the gods", i.e. of the fundamental principles and symbols.
>   (C.G.Jung, The Undiscovered Self, 1958 - in [1]).

Since the earliest times, dreams have been used in various cultures, from ancient Greece to Egypt, from Native Americans to Africa and Australia, as a common way of reliving the past, learning from the present, orienting the future.

That dreams can have a "social function," i.e., be influenced and in turn influence the context in which we live is therefore nothing new. On the contrary, we could say that it is a very old idea, which in many cultures has been for centuries, and is still today, considered a source of wisdom for the entire community.

Psychoanalysis at the beginning of the last century highly contributed to restore the central role of dreams in our experience of reality. Ever since Freud defined the dream as the "royal road to the unconscious," [2] dreams have become a window on another world, an inner, hidden world whose latent message is difficult for the dreamer to comprehend, but which it is possible to decode through analysis.

The manifest content of the dream, according to Freud, appears as a "hodge-podge of meanings" that mixes undesirable psychic fragments, repressed ancient memories and residues of daytime reality; a sort of "temporary psychosis" whose interpretation in a psychoanalytic key is the translation and recomposition of the dream in waking reality. The dreamworld is thus an "other" world, partly alien to waking life, with which it comes into conflict if it is not brought back to it through interpretation. Hillman writes in this regard:

> Now the contours of the conflict loom clearly: on the one hand, the dream belongs completely to sleep; on the other, interpretation must bring the dream back into the daytime

E. Pasini, C. Trimboli, *A Social Dreaming Experience at the Time of COVID 19*, New Paradigms in Healthcare, https://doi.org/10.1007/978-3-031-42498-4_4

world, rescuing it, let us say, or 'redeeming' it (according to Freud's metaphor) from its
infernal madness and immersion in the pleasure principle.
   [3, p. 24]

Freud, however, by emphasizing the personal significance of dreams and the unconscious as the realm of the repressed "locked dreams in a room," the room of analysis, and made it a land of conquest over which the ego can little by little expand its
conscious control over reality.

The social function of dreams, the subject of this investigation, therefore seems
to have got lost along the way, hidden behind a myriad of individual stories that are
difficult to trace back to a collective meaning. In this chapter I will therefore attempt
to follow the traces of the social function of the dream by going back in time and
space, to describe some of its manifestations as they have been expressed by different cultures of the past and distant present, using the idea developed by Jung of the
collective unconscious.

We live in an era of profound transformations, in which it is increasingly evident
that the patterns of thinking that we have used so far, and that have sustained the
Western culture for centuries, seem to have stopped working.

In the last 3 years, the global pandemic of COVID-19, the climate crisis, international social and economic conflicts, the long lasting war between Russia and Ukraine
have paved the way for fears that were already in the air, namely that our social system could be no longer sustainable in the long term. The "end of history," which
some had coincided with the establishment of the liberal capitalist system as the best
of all possible worlds, seems to have suddenly turned into an apocalyptic nightmare.

Today we are trying to adjust to the idea that our life system has to be changed
before coming to an end, but face to this possibility we are bereft of viable
alternatives.

Our relationships with nature, time, duration, history have lost their meaning
behind the impetus of opposing tensions that seem to be driven by ungovernable forces.

Internal tensions explode in a fragmented, anomic social context, where inequalities and unease become increasingly visible.

In lack of a common purpose, individuals act like crazed splinters, totally
immersed in a cacophonous multimedia universe that transmits only virtual simulacra of fake images.

Alongside the unease, however, signs of the need to recover the sense of a collective "we" are arising, in order to identify, together, viable alternatives.

The Italian Listening Post session held in Milan in January 2023 as part of the
international observatory on psychosocial trends highlighted the misalignment
between major social issues (pandemic, war, climate crisis) that collectively we are
no longer able to manage, and individual behaviors, which are swinging between
"autistic isolation" and "compulsive sociability," two opposing tensions that have
increased during the pandemic as symptom of a profound social malaise. Faced
with an increasingly threatening external reality, states and governments react in a
disorganized, paranoid, meaningless manner. The idea that we have lost a sense of
"we," of togetherness, is enhanced, together with the fear that there is not even the
vaguest idea of what could be done to build a new one.

Yet, "flowers can be born from rubble", as underlined by the metaphor that ended the 2023 International Listening Post session in Milan. To this end, face of such a destructive reality the collective dimension of "new us" may be far away to come, but everyone is called upon to play her own responsibility, as a necessity for our very survival.

Could the complex messages that dreams conceal, which go beyond the limited reality of individual experience, help us to recompose our broken relationship with the world, reviving common feelings and founding a new idea of community, which are indispensable to deal with the disruptive dimensions of the many collective traumas we are facing today?

To retrace the social function of the dreams, that was very much alive in many cultures of the past and also at the present time, we will take a glance of some few examples of how dreams could be a stimulus to move away from a one-dimensional vision of reality, and an opening toward a multiplicity of different worlds, which is essential today if we want to have a chance to imagine our future in an ever-changing reality.

The exploration of the social function of dreams starts from ancient Greece, the cradle of the mythological thought that founded the Western psyche in its historical tradition.

In ancient Greece, and later in Rome, dreams were considered a key to predict the future.

The Greeks believed in fact that dreams "came from afar" and provided clues that could often be surprising or disconcerting, but never gave clear answers.

Dreams consisted of images, *eidola*, forms and figures from the world of ideas that could be seen in dreams as reflected shadows of reality. Such premonitory dreams with powerful symbolic and prophetic content could be told, shared, and passed down from generation to generation to celebrate the fame, plots, and destinies of heroes and gods.

The Iliad, for instance, recounts the famous Achilles' dream, when the Greek hero was visited in sleep by the shadow of Patroclus who asked him for a honorable burial so that he could find peace in Hades; and the deceptive dream of Agamemnon, who was promised a victory in battle, that brought instead the Achaeans close to defeat.

Again in the Iliad, Hector's death is described as a dreamlike prophetic tale repeated ad infinitum, where since the beginning we are aware of the unfortunate destiny the gods decided for the Trojan hero, who is the scapegoat chased by Achilles all the way to the walls of Troy, with no chance to escape.

In ancient Greece, therefore, dreams could be deceptive and treacherous, but they always had something important to reveal and should be listened to, because they showed a new perspective on reality that, if ignored, could prove to be fatal.

This way of dealing with dreams highlighted the deep connection of the dreamworld with the realm of the shadow and the world of the dead. The real world was considered a pale reflection of the underworld, in a "dramatic reversal" between the two worlds, the supernal world of wakefulness and the subterranean world of dreams.

Dream images were therefore, as Hillmann suggested, expressions of the underworld, similar to the "mundus imaginalis" described by Henry Corbin, and could not be reduced to mere representations of individual inner realities. In this perspective mythology can be seen as a true "psychology of images," the contact bridge between the upper world and the underworld, between life and death.

Today, the deep connection between these two worlds is lost, and behind the clear-cut separation between life and death lies the refusal to recognize, and the incapacity to integrate, the existence of the underworld. This loss of contact with "the world of the threshold" separates us from the dreamlike reality of the shadow, but at the same time puts us at its mercy. A rupture that was evident in the profound laceration we have experienced today, due to the lack of rituals for a collective mourning of the many deaths caused by the pandemic.

The Greek art of healing had thoroughly explored this boundary, giving a great relevance to dreams in the purification rituals propaedeutical to the therapeutic process of the cult of Asclepius, the god of Medicine. The dreams that ritually took place in the temple of Apollo were a source of visions through which the gods or goddesses manifested their voice and showed the sick person the way to healing.

Moving from Ancient Greece to Egypt, the Egyptian art of divination also attached great importance to dreams.

In ancient Egypt, dreams were divided into "good dreams," the source of which was the god Horus, and "bad dreams," that came from the god Set and were considered nightmares, filled with entities that tormented the sleeper. In ancient Egypt one did not say "having a dream," as the dream was not an action, but instead "seeing a dream" or "seeing something in a dream," thus acknowledging the existence of a phenomenon external to the sleeper. Even in ancient Egypt, therefore, the dream was understood as a link between two different worlds, the human and the afterlife world, the latter inhabited by the gods and the shadows of the dead. Dreams occupied a kind of "liminal space" on the border with the afterworld, in which the entities that inhabited it were only partially visible and attainable. The underworld was the inverse of the diurnal world, an inverted world in which the dead walked upside down, populated by a multiplicity of forms, each of them partial representation of the whole person.

The dream thus restored a sense of multiplicity, ideally representing the impossibility of thinking of a finite undivided individuality and giving wings to the infinity of the soul.

In the Bible the dream is considered instead rather as a "revelation," the instrument for God to communicate with his prophets.

In the Old Testament the most famous biblical dreamers include Joseph, whose ability to interpret dreams won him the favor of the Pharaoh of Egypt, overcoming the jealousy and the traps of his brothers; King Solomon owed his famous wisdom to dreams; and Jacob was revealed of the divine benevolence in a dream.

In the biblical narrative, however, the revelatory dream is not attainable to all but is reserved to some chosen few, as a gift of the divine grace that always seems to require a certain discernment, and the sacred texts warn against the false prophets who "see the false and give vain consolations, leading people away from God." Not everyone is able to hear and interpret the language of dreams and the divine word establishes a clear hierarchy between those who are truly authorized to do so and those who are not.

Following the traces of dreams in cultures historically considered "primitive," the Australian Aboriginal tradition place the boundaries between the dreamworld and the real world in a very thin, practically non-existent, borderline space.

Bruce Chatwin recounts in his book *The Songlines [4]* that for the Australian Aborigines, the land is marked by an interweaving of "dream tracks," a labyrinth of paths visible only to their eyes that were formed by the "footprints of the Ancestors" who had "dreamt the world" of the beginning. The Time of Dreaming is therefore a mythical time-place zone, the spatial and temporal dimension where the ancestral spirits of the creators "sang the world" and gave rise to the "sound" arrangement of a formless cosmos.

The Australian Aboriginal mythology recounts that the original displacements of people into the chaotic primordial world took place in the dream dimension, a mythical time still sung about today through the stories and music that accompany the periodic displacements of the nomadic peoples of the inland Australia. The "walkabout" of the Australian Aborigines, a pilgrimage that each individual does during the course of his or her lifetime in order to reach the original creative center at the source of being, is an initiatory journey behind which lies a veritable "metaphysics of nomadism," together with an artistic and ecological culture that is as enigmatic, sophisticated and fascinating to the Western eyes as ever, despite the material scarcity in which these peoples still live today. In the Time of Dreaming nature and culture coincide, and the dream is the tangible, physical and psychic manifestation of this profound unity. In the walkabout everyone "sings the world," repeating the words and music of the ancestors at the moment of creation, and in doing so it is as if, each time, they "recreate the world" starting from a center, the center of the person and at the same time the center of all.

In the American Indian cultures, the dream is a vision that has deep cultural roots, playing an important role in preserving the traditions of the origins from the oppression of the white man. The Native Americans consider dreams gateways to invisible realities; they are not the prerogative of individuals, far from it, but an access potentially open to all that can be entered to show the reality of the imaginal world that lies beyond the sensible experience. It is a world populated by animals and spirits that in the dream manifest themselves in human forms, inner expressions with which it is nevertheless possible to establish a profound relationship of similarity and otherness. The way of dreaming and visioning is therefore open to all and is considered a master of life; but for this to happen there are certain figures, the shamans, who act as intermediaries between their community and the parallel world of dreams. "Specialists in ecstasy," shamans are repositories of knowledge, tools, practices, stories, ritual dances, through which it is possible to convey the passage between the two worlds, while preserving their original essence.

The "dreamcatcher," a small object of daily use among the Native Americans which is now popular all over the world, is a good example of the profound intertwining between everyday life and complex symbolic contents. Symbol of the Native American heritage, the dreamcatcher has the function of capturing nefarious dreams before they enter the sleeper's psyche, expressing the indigenous conception that dreams are sent from the outside, for the most varied reasons, and do not originate from inside the dreamer. Dreams are not therefore products of the psyche, but rather it is the psyche itself that acts as a "receiving antenna" for messages that come from elsewhere, and the journey between these two worlds can also be facilitated with the help of psychotropic substances that open up to complex imaginative experiences. This leads to the construction of a true "art of dreaming," such as described by Carlos Castaneda in his encounters with Don Juan and the "peyote culture." [5]

Finally, to conclude our dream journey, it is worth mentioning the practice of the collective use of dreams made by the Senoi, an indigenous population of the interior of Malaysia, who made of dream-telling the foundation of their political, social, and educational order. The Senoi, says Morton Schatzman in his wide work of investigation, use dream-telling at different levels and in different public and private situations.

Since childhood they learn to dream together and to share their dreams in the community gatherings and within the family. Once "dreamed together," the dreams become resources for the entire community, for the discovery of the inner potential of the individuals and the group which is much needed to overcome difficult impasses. Due to their customs of sharing of dreams the Senoi, despite their poor material living conditions, have become a much-quoted example of an almost perfect social equilibrium. Their society is free of violent crimes, armed conflicts, mental and physical illnesses; their example, although small and marginal, reminds us of how in some social contexts the dream was considered and was treated from the outset, as a "social object," able to create, recreate, and transform social relationships, thus giving life to intercultural and intergenerational bonds that are able to "last over time."

4.2 Gordon Lawrence and the Origin of Social Dreaming

We saw in the previous paragraph how dreams, among many cultures of the past and many indigenous peoples, have always been treated as a source of wisdom, and how the images that appear in dreams often refer to collective patterns that feed the imagination and at the same time provide content for shared foundations, origins, behaviors. Social Dreaming draws on the anthropological tradition of cross-cultural comparisons, revisited through the eyes and lifelong experience of its "discoverer," the British psychoanalyst Gordon Lawrence, who highlighted features and meanings of dream sharing that are of the highest relevance today.

Social Dreaming originated and was initially pioneered by its founder Gordon Lawrence in the early 1980s, in the cultural milieu of the Tavistock Institute for Human Relations in London. At the beginning of the 1970s Gordon Lawrence was one of the most prominent representatives of the Tavistock, whose international reputation is linked to pioneering work in the analysis of group dynamics and leadership mechanisms within organizations. The Tavistock methodology has its roots in the sociodynamic school of Human Relations of Elton Mayo and Kurt Lewin and in the psychoanalytic clinical approach. At the Tavistock Clinic Wilfred Bion, during and immediately after World War II, began his group work with patients who had undergone highly traumatic experiences during the conflict.

For over 10 years, Gordon Lawrence worked at the Tavistock to develop the prestigious Leicester Conference, from which the Tavistock methodology of working with groups originated. In the mid-1980s, following a troubled career choice, Lawrence left the Tavistock and founded the Social Dreaming school.

As extensively analyzed in the introduction of this book (see chapter 1 - Introduction to Social Dreaming) Social Dreaming stems from Lawrence's psychoanalytic background and from his work experiences in groups but overturns one of the main dogmas of classical psychoanalysis, suggesting a choral way of sharing dreams where the focus is on the dream and not on the dreamer.

I had the chance to meet Gordon Lawrence for the first time in the summer of 2006.

I was writing at the time a book on charisma, and I was deeply intrigued by the complex relationship between the leader and his/her follower, that seemed to me lying somewhere in a sort of middle earth, in between the individual and the collective space.

In such a liminal space the strong projections the followers make onto the charismatic leader seem to be grounded on a powerful shared imaginary. I did not know much about Social Dreaming at that time, but the little I knew made me think that it could have been an extraordinary opportunity to explore the most hidden aspects of the charismatic phenomenon, which were the main crux of my search: the investigation of the connections between individual imagination and collective imaginary.

I met Gordon Lawrence for a conversation on charisma in his house at Hampstead Heath, in the Northern part of London, on a summer afternoon in August 2006.

The magic atmosphere of his studio, full of books, carpets, and paintings, some of them his own work, the many objects he had got from his travels all around the world, but most of all Lawrence eclectic personality, contributed to add a particular charm to our encounter, an almost magical intensity to our conversation. Reporting integrally some passages of it is the better way, I believe, to highlight how Social Dreaming was conceived and put to work from the living voice of its founder.

The extract is taken from my book *Carisma, il segreto del leader (Charisma, the leader's secret),* published by Garzanti, Milano, 2009, by courtesy of the editor.

Gordon Lawrence. I joined the Tavistock in 1971, at the age of 38, and my collaboration lasted until the mid-80s. The idea of Social Dreaming was born from group experiences. I had noticed that in meetings, when a dream was offered to the group, it was always illuminating. This reflection intrigued me a lot, and I wondered what would have happened if we had adopted a different perspective on dreams, a sociocentric perspective instead of an egocentric one, which is the one with which dreams have been used for centuries. When the Leicester Conference was established to explore the unconscious in relation to leadership, I wondered why we couldn't explicitly use dreams for the exploration. I did a lot of research on my own, but I couldn't give a coherent shape to the idea. Social Dreaming was the last thing I did at Tavistock. I had been thinking about social dreams for years and couldn't quite fit it together, and then I read Charlotte Berardt's book The Third Reich Dreams [6], and bang!!... everything clipped together. I was profoundly inspired by that book. Beradt was a German journalist who in the 1930s had collected the dreams of some Jews, and from their analysis it was clear that they could not only be the product of an unresolved inner conflict but came from the social context of Nazi Germany. The dreams that Beradt told were based on the persecution of the Jews, on fears and lies that were in the air and constituted a real threat. The idea of the context as the source of dreams was new to me, but I felt that it could be the basis of Social Dreaming; and then I began to develop this idea. In February 1982, I conducted the first Social Dreaming Matrix experiment, and left Tavistock in March of that year. Three years later I was invited to a conference in Israel, and on that occasion I first used the name of Social Dreaming and the model I still use today.

Elisabetta Pasini. Could we say that your work on Social Dreaming, the school you have created and the new way to look at dreams are the result of a life change, stem from your decision to leave the Tavistock and start your own personal journey? That Social Dreaming was born from a moment of transition in life, that was also rather painful and difficult, I believe.

GL. In some ways it is. After leaving the Tavistock I went through a period of deep depression, which nevertheless was very productive for me, although I have often thought that those ten years were the worst time of my life and I would not want to go through it all again. However, despite everything, I had to find a way to live, to support my family, and I had to devise a system to overcome the disappointment. Sometimes it is precisely the circumstances in which you find yourself that force you to look at things in a new way. I started writing because in the circumstances I was in I felt I had to do it, leaving the Tavistock forced me to work hard on Social Dreaming; even if, since the beginning of my activity as an analyst, I have always tried to question the dogmas I had learned about dreams by asking myself what they could tell us about life in society.

Throughout my life I have never followed the ideas of the majority, I have never belonged to any establishment, and I think that you can only get close to the new if you don't belong to an establishment. In fact, I believe that creative ideas have a different origin from that associated with purpose-oriented activities, and in this regard it's important to remember what Donald Winnicott wrote about the transitional space, that space in which psychological phenomena are formed that are "not me". It's easy to be a rebellious teenager, but what I have always tried to do is to question what seemed obvious, I think I have been like this since I was a child ... When the war broke out in 1939, I was five years old and was sent to staying with my grandparents who lived in the countryside, and I lived with them for three years. That was one of the best times of my life: I could do pretty much anything I wanted, go anywhere and explore the space around me with very few limits, apart from being at home for lunch time and a few other fixed rules. It was a very formative experience, one of the best experiences I've ever had, and I told about it in Roots in a Northern Landscape [7]. I certainly idealized this experience, perhaps beyond what it actually was, but I am sure it was there that I learned to be alone with my thoughts. I have often wondered if the seeds of the idea of Social Dreaming had not been sown in that period. One of my favorite games, then, was building forts with old rubber tires that were in my grandparents' yard…. Social Dreaming maybe also comes from this experience, because somehow it has to do with "rearranging the furniture of the world" so that it takes on a different configuration, a different sequence, just like a good painter does with his art. The great painters reconfigure the world continuously. Creativity simply happens, it's above all a fact of luck and synchrony, not a logical process. Some ideas may not be good, this is true, and ultimately must be discarded, but nevertheless one must always look forward; even if, from time to time, you feel depressed. I am a big advocate of depression, nothing new can come about if you don't go through bouts of depression. Being depressed means touching what it really means to be human, accepting the tragic component of life. Who is never depressed, who is always happy and full of life, lives an empty life, in a false world, just follows the group; because people tend to simplify. To become something you are not, you have to experience destructiveness in your inner world. Wasn't it Joseph Conrad talking about sailing on the edge of destruction?

The bad thing is that many use Social Dreaming for their own personal narcissistic ends, while I try to follow the idea of losing one's ego in the Matrix, abandoning purpose-oriented actions in order to see reality with other eyes through the dreams. [8, p. 102–104]

4.3   Social Dreaming and Transformative Thinking

"Social Dreaming has to do with rearranging the furniture of the world, so that it takes on a different configuration, a different sequence, just like a good painter does with his art," said Gordon Lawrence in the conversation reported above. I always liked this metaphor, that highlights how in the matrix offering a dream to the group is a gift that, through the associations and amplifications made by others, opens up to the possibility of discovering new aspects of the reality we are immersed on.

The experience of Social Dreaming is like an undulatory movement of constant oscillation between the inside and the outside, in which shreds of dreams are used as pieces of a mosaic to compose a canvas of possible meanings, that does not interpret though but combine, creates concatenations of elements, strengthens relationships.

Sharing a dream in a safe and protected space such as the Matrix gives space to an imaginative and narrative function that reconnects to an enormous wealth of knowledge, fantasies, myths, stories, collective narratives, everything that characterizes us as human beings, from which derives all the potential of Social Dreaming.

Sharing dreams allows to connect with others and to differentiate from them, to mirror ourselves in others and to measure the distance that separates from them. In the Social Dreaming Matrix we can experience the "psychic space of the threshold" that lies in the "middle earth" between the individual and the collective. Which is, I argue, the first step to give rise to a "transformative thinking."

To better explore the hypothesis that Social Dreaming favors the development of a transformative thinking, I would like to take into consideration the three forms of thinking, magical thinking, oneiric thinking, transformative thinking, described by T.H.Ogden in his book Reclaiming Unlived Lives (Vite non vissute, [9]).[1]

Ogden defines magical thinking as a kind of anti-thinking in which the subject is unable to deal with the connection between internal and external reality and develops fantasies of omnipotence aimed at replacing actual reality with an invented one. Inevitably solipsistic, magical thinking is driven by the projection of emotions the subjects feels unbearable into the external world, that lead to the denial of the experience of the others as someone different from myself. The incapacity to find a boundary between what is "me and not-me," leads to a one sided magical thinking that seriously undermines relationships with a progressive deterioration of the capacity for symbolization. There is no need to emphasize how widespread this form of thinking is today, making itself visible in many social media chat and forums that provide tons of examples of magical thinking!

The oneiric thinking, on the other hand, pertains to the area of dreams and reveries. Like dreamlike fantasies that goes on even during the waking time, the oneiric thinking ushers to a rich and nonlinear area of thoughts, that, through imagination, allows the subject to look at the daily experience from a variety of points of view giving rise to psychological growth. Ogden defines it as

---

[1]The following quotes are taken from the Italian version of Ogden's book Reclaiming Unlived Lives, Vite non vissute, Cortina, 2016. The translation in English from the Italian version is mine.

dreaming thought without the awareness of its destination, only carried away by its movement. [9, p. 38]

The transformative thinking marks instead the access to a different order of thought, defined as

> a form of oneiric thinking that implies the recognition of the limits of the categories of meaning that are usually thought to be the only possible ones ... and the creation in substitution of fundamentally new categories - a radically new way of organizing the experience - which up to that point were unimaginable. [9, p. 40]

And again:

> The psychological shift of one's Gestalt (conceptual / experiential) inherent in transformative thinking creates the potential for types of feelings, forms of object relationship and quality of being alive that the individual had never experienced before. This type of thinking always requires the minds of at least two people, since the isolated individual cannot radically change the fundamental categories of meaning with which he organizes his experience. [9, p. 42].

To give an example of transformative thinking, Ogden takes the parable of Christ and the adulteress. Jesus Christ, when asked about the law that requires the sinner adulteress to be stoned to death, replies: "Let those of you who are without sin cast the first stone". Jesus does not give a direct answer, however, but moves the question to another level. Before speaking, Jesus takes a long pause for reflection and writes something with his finger in the sand. What he wrote we will never know, but it is important to underline how, rather than giving a direct answer, Jesus opens up to a different psychological space, that of writing, which also becomes a new space of thought, from which new questions arise. "Let those of you who are without sin cast the first stone" in fact is not an answer, but opens to new questions that interrogate individual responsibility, social conformity, and the same category of sin. Transformative thinking therefore implies the recognition of the limits of the usual categories of thought and the creation of fundamentally new categories, by moving to different cognitive registers and the use of different languages that, beyond words, activate the imagination.

Transformative thinking arises therefore from a plurality of minds. Looking into themselves and the recognition and acceptance of the other open up to a new world of possibilities, capable to bring together multiple points of view and to imagine different facets of reality.

Imagination can be seen in this process as a way to broaden the one-sided narrow views of the ego defenses, inevitably limited because constantly seeking compromises to adapt to reality, pushing one to venture onto the rugged terrain of self-expansion.

Transformative thinking develops the ability to focus on aspects not yet clearly understood at a conscious level, in a way that is both "reflexive" (looking at one's inner world with an introverted vision) and "satellite" (looking outwards with an extroverted look), allowing the discovery of new perspectives and enhancing the sharing of a social imaginary.

For this to happen, however, we need a specific setting as a safe and good container of the experience. The Social Dreaming Matrix, I argue, is such a container.

The term Matrix is an ambiguous term: on the one hand it has been used since the beginning, and must be understood, in its literal meaning of womb, incubator, an intermediate generative space in which something new can happen.

On the other hand, "matrix" also refers to "the matrix of the undifferentiated unconscious," a potentially threatening and chaotic space in which the mind could easily get lost. Which reminds us to the importance of emphasizing, once more, that the focus of Social Dreaming is on the dream and not on the dreamer. Because only the certainty that a dream, once given to the group, can be taken up by all as part of a creative experience in a safe and secure space, guarantees that, through the images of dreams, a transformation may occur.

"Leaving your Ego out the door," as Gordon Lawrence wished and as the host of the matrix always suggests at the beginning of the experience, requires therefore to rely on, and allow ourself to indulge, a transitional space; which is not, however, the regressive return to the mother's womb, nor the frightening loss of the Self into a chaotic space.

Rather, it is the "dreamtime" of the Australian aborigines, or the web of threads and feathers of which the "dreamcatchers" of the Native Americans are made; it is a time that opens up to a potentially infinite space, thinkable because is safely shared and contained.

> While we are conscious, we are highly self-reflective, making use of the "I", or the ego, to think through our experience; but in dreaming we are not "egocentric" for the "I" is less important as we lose ourselves in the "thereness" of the dream. [10, p. 7]

Ultimately, the matrix is not a group experience, and it is important to emphasize the difference, because a group is an organism characterized by a system of roles, with a dynamic that tends to repeat and reproduce itself with recognizable and interpretable patterns of behavior, whereas the matrix is a potentially generative space in which new meanings are created, in order to understand the changes we are experiencing and how we can deal with them.

Today we tend to define the reality in which we live as a fluid reality, in which change is constantly occurring before our eyes; often, however, we feel overwhelmed by the speed of change, we feel we lack the tools and means to process and metabolize it.

Today, we have lot of contents, but few containers to process the experience of change. Which is why, in my opinion, Social Dreaming is such a valuable experience.

Because, despite all the time we spend surfing the social networks to give visibility and resonance to our opinions, what we really lack are real spaces of free thinking that could help us to walk toward the future.

The dreaming space of the matrix is a synchronic space, a space, as Jung said, of "meaningful coincidences" not necessarily ordered by a cause–effect relationship. In the matrix we leave the comfort zone of the rational empirical thought and enter into a universe of synchronic a-causal connections, a "multiverse" of meanings that opens up to infinite possibilities of transformation.

> Social Dreaming accepts synchronicity. In a Social Dreaming Matrix, where the dreams come from infinite sets of the unconscious, it is possible to work out connections and links between the dreams which are not apparently causally related. One hypothesis, for exam-

ple, is that the very first dream of a Matrix is a fractal of all the dreams that are to follow. Free associations give this fractal more substance. [10, p. 11]

4.4   The Analytical Psychology of C.G. Jung

The Analytical Psychology of C.G.Jung has always interwoven a close relationship with the "interstices of reality," intermediate zones in which many "borderline phenomena" dwell. Those phenomena occur in the thin threshold that separates, and at the same time connects, the individual and the collective realms and can be explored through the technique of Active Imagination, a way of consciously access the creative potential of the unconscious through the amplification of dreams, images, narratives, drawings, reveries. Conceived by Jung in the *Red Book* as an imaginative process, Active Imagination takes the dreams in a "prospective" way, amplifying and visualizing them through symbols, images and narratives in order to bridge the conscious ego with unconscious contents.

> Every good idea and all creative work are the offspring of imagination. …The debt we owe to the play of imagination is incalculable. (C.G. Jung, CW 6, §93.)

In the long journey of exploration of the unconscious described in the Red Book, Jung portrays his discovery and dialogues with his own internal characters as a narrative, in which the encounter with the dark side is often painful, difficult, develops in harsh desert soils, interspersed with dark nights and long silences.

His journey, however, is not a solitary one, because the main discovery, and the greatest adventure, is to realize that the characters he meets along the way are not just his own fantasies but belong to a much wider reality populated by archetypes, collective images, dreams.

A dense network of myths, stories, and narratives, says Jung [11], connects each individual existence to an enormously larger world in which one can recognize and experience one's own difference and uniqueness, following his/her process of individuation.

> The hypothesis of a collective unconscious belongs to the class of ideas that people at first find strange but soon come to possess and use as familiar conceptions. (C.G. Jung, CW9-1, Archetype of the Collective Unconscious, §1)

The idea of the collective unconscious is possibly one of the main contributions Jung gave to the deep psychology and to the entire story of the human thinking.

While Freud's unconscious was exclusively personal, Jung added to the personal unconscious—which contents are the complexes that represent the personal part of the psychic life—the idea of the collective unconscious, an inborn, universal, common psyche which contents are the archetypes. Universal images that pertain to the whole mankind since the most remote time of the species, archetypes' conscious representations can be traced through myths, fairy tales, and stories all along the different cultures.

However, the whole meaning of the archetypes can never be fully grasped, because, as integral part of the unconscious, they are only partially accessible to the human mind, through hints, small bits of experience attainable in dreams, embodying the connection between matter and mind. We could therefore say that archetypes are symbolic expressions of an inner psyche, mainly experienced as projections of external phenomena, which stand at the basis of the unique experience of divine that gives a numinous sense to the human existence.

Jung speaks of a "mythopoeic level of the Psyche," in which what he called the "fantastic associative thought" supports through images, the function of "mythical creation" of the unconscious, that we experience as a sort of connection with the transcendent. An experience, however, we are not able to entirely grasp, to fully embrace, but we can feel it exists, not only on a metaphysical level but also within us. It is the level of the archetypal universal structures, which always possess, nevertheless, a certain degree of ambiguity; because they are, at the same time, compelling patterns of repetitive actions without an evident consistency of meaning—like the archetypal characters that we find in fairy tales, in example—and abstract ideas that remain detached from action, at the platonic level of purely intellectual speculation. It is through imagination and the symbolic function that we can put together "what is inside"—a learned behavior, an emotion, an intuition—with "what is outside," leading back to a pregnancy of meaning. Because the images are not only representations, they are dynamic principles that convey many complex imaginative experiences.

> Symbols are not signs or allegories for something known; they seek rather to express something that is little known or completely unknown. (C.G. Jung, Symbols of Transformation, CW5, §329)

Symbols are "active agents of change" that point to unconscious details, disclose different perspectives, unlock apparently closed doors; they draw our attention to unexpected meanings that resonate in us transcending their contents. While preserving their mystery, symbols disclose glimpses of possible discoveries, their emotional force expressing the dynamic power of an archetype represented in the form of an image. As Neumann said [12],

> Symbols constitute the openly visible aspects of the archetype, that correspond to its latent invisibility. While in the primordial archetype the most various symbols, which the conscious mind sees as contrasting, coexist, they separate later and organize themselves following the opposites principle. Like the archetype, symbols have a dynamic and a content component... The symbol therefore, leaving aside its dynamic effect of "energy transformer", is also a "conscience molder", pushing the psyche to process the conscious and unconscious contents included in it. [12, p. 57]

A symbol points, brings tension and movements to an archetype in connection to a specific moment and situation in time. Symbols work, therefore, as "thinking in movement," pushing the conscience to process meanings and feelings; they work at an imaginative level, making accessible different aspects of reality. When an archetype becomes visible by the conscious mind, is because at this moment the unconscious meets consciousness.

Jung says that this idea was pretty clear for the primitive men, who were not looking for objective rational explanations of the natural phenomena, but were open instead to find correspondences between the inner and the outer experience of the world. The inner experience of a numinous self in close contact with the divine forces of nature was the essence of the primitive mind; the danger of "loosing the soul," the individual struggle once the collective experience of a whole superior totality is lost was one of the deepest fears of the primitive men. Modern men, Jung says, have lost this connection with the symbolic experience of the world. The development in the last centuries of the rational scientific explanation of the world stated the ultimate separation of the modern man from a deep connection between matter and psyche. Psychology as the new science of the psyche, instead of helping to renew this bond, focused on the individual experience and on the prevalence of the I/You relationship, which ultimately leads to an infinite fragmentation of projections, an inflation of meaningless representations of the world. But, we should ask ourselves, what is in the long run the meaning of this impoverishment of symbols? Where are we leaded to, if the human capacity to represent the "struggles of the soul" is constantly undermined by the lack of "collective representations," those parts of the collective unconscious that have been consciously elaborated?

We can no longer avoid the confrontation with the unconscious and its archetypal contents, letting them free to outgrow unseen and unbridled.

However, a head-on encounter with the unconscious is never a good idea, especially when it comes to a potentially traumatic psychic reality, which is a source of intolerable suffering against which over time the conscious ego raises powerful defenses, necessary for its psychic survival. Face to a traumatic experience, the crossing of the threshold is impossible. In the encounter with the archetypal world we should be able therefore to develop a "lateral sight," a point of view that makes us capable to look at things in a different way, allowing to tackle the unconscious parts from a lateral, indirect perspective. Activating a lateral sight is not therefore only a strategy to get around the obstacle but is a way to bring out unexpected inner resources, in a space of wider possibilities where a greater self-awareness can slowly creep in and grow.

As M.L.Von Franz pointed out [13], in the darkest night, a fable flame is better than the dazzling, blinding light of the sun:

> If clarity of consciousness is too strong it has a destructive aspect. It burns all those mysterious archetypal processes that cannot be pulled into the realm of collective consciousness. Every person who is in the way of individuation will discover, in some form, the necessity of keeping certain things entirely to himself... There are things not even discussed with oneself – they must be left in the twilight and must not be looked at too exactly. There are secret things of the soul that can only grow in the dark – the clear sun of consciousness burns their life away. [13, p. 104]

We could call this side-look with different names, which refer to different possibilities of activation. It is Winnicott's "transitional space," a protected space of play and containment where is possible to experience the difference between "what is me and not me." It is Campbell's "hero's journey," the mythical structure of an initiatory path of transformation and individuation.

The side view we want to underline in this work is our experience of Social Dreaming at the time of COVID-19: a journey of exploration and amplification of dreams and narratives that, in the face of the highly traumatic upheaval that the

COVID-19 pandemic brought into our lives, made us more aware of those night-mares and fears that had gone unheeded for too long, revealing the fragility and powerlessness of our contemporary society.

Together with the deep sense of loss and discouragement we all felt during the pandemic, however, an urgent, unexpected need to explore different ways of living emerged, a desire to find out new connections between our individual destinies and our need for collective meanings. As if only a lateral shift could help to bring to life an "expectation of the extraordinary" in the present, the pandemic conceived the feeble awareness that to recover a common future we had to accept to finally face the ghosts and fears that had been removed for too long.

The etymology of the word symbol derives from the Greek "symballo," meaning to unite, to hold together.

The space of the symbolic is therefore an epistemological terrain of thinking that does not ground only on opposition and contrast, but on the capacity to connect, held together, opposing elements. It is the territory of the unity of the multiple, which anticipates the possibility of creating new worlds.

References

1. Graeber D, Wengrow D. The dawn of everything. New York: Penguin Books; 2021.
2. Freud S. L'Interpretazione dei Sogni. Roma: Newton Compton; 1970.
3. Hillman J. Il sogno e il mondo infero. Milano: Adelphi; 1979.
4. Chatwin B, Le Vie dei Canti. Milano: Adelphi; 1988.
5. Castaneda C. A Scuola dallo Stregone. Roma: Astrolabio; 1968.
6. Beradt C. Il Terzo Reich dei Sogni. Milano: Meltemi Press; 2020.
7. Lawrence G. Tongued with fire. London: Karnac books; 2000.
8. Pasini E, Natili F. Carisma, il segreto del leader. Milano: Garzanti; 2009.
9. Ogden TH. Vite non vissute. Milano: Cortina; 2016.
10. Lawrence G. Infinite possibilities of social dreaming. London: Karnac Books; 2007.
11. Jung CG. The archetypes of the collective unconscious, CW9–1. Princeton University Press; 1959.
12. Neumann E. La grande madre. Roma: Astrolabio; 1974.
13. Von Franz ML. The feminine in fairytales. Boston: Shambala; 1993.

Chapter 5
The Narrative and Semiotic Approach

5.1 The Narrative Function: From the Origins to the Studies in Social Sciences

Telling and hearing stories is a fundamental need inherent in human nature that has been debated since the earliest times.

Already in ancient Greece Plato and Aristotle agreed that art was due to our natural predisposition for representational imitation (*mimesis*) and that this willingness to understand the world was a distinctive element of our human species in comparison with other animals. But if Plato condemned poetry, especially drama, seen as the representation and exaltation of harmful passions, Aristotle, in his work "Poetics," [1] argued that tragedy precisely induced a positive effect in spectators. Aristotle thus highlights the social and psychological function of art. According to Aristotle, not only do we have a natural predisposition in imitating, but there is also a connotation of pleasure inherent in it: the intense emotional experience we experience through aesthetic contemplation or literary works, described as *catharsis*, allows purification from passions and produces a beneficial effect on the person.

According to Aristotle, among the elements of drama, there is one that is by far the most important of all and that is the "*mythos*," what we might translate as plot. The *mythos* has to do with the composition of facts. And therein lies the sensemaking function of narratives. Plot represents the essence of storytelling, it is what binds the content together and makes a story compelling. Its purpose, therefore, is to produce meaning. Aristotle's *mythos* is about action (physical and psychological). It uses people, objectives and obstacles, conflicts, complications, reversals, and acknowledgments to create a state of empathy on the part of the viewer, creating intense experiences of fear and pity until reaching catharsis and relief. Introducing an order, placing events within a storyline, makes it possible to cope with the

E. Pasini, C. Trimboli, *A Social Dreaming Experience at the Time of COVID 19*, New Paradigms in Healthcare, https://doi.org/10.1007/978-3-031-42498-4_5

chaotic mass of experiences and perceptions that increasingly characterize the lives of individuals [2, 3].

There are many studies and reflections that have developed over time successively to Aristotle's first enlightening ideas, but it is in the twentieth century that theories and models that study and reflect on the function of narratives were first developed.

Vladimir Propp, in the early 1900s is one of the first major modern authors to deal with storytelling. Linguist and anthropologist, in his work "Morphology of the Fairy Tale" [4] he analyzes the structure of a hundred traditional Russian fairy tales. It is the first work that studies fairy tales as a narrative product and identifies in them precise rules in the structure of the tale, with constant characters and patterns that are repeated.

Getting lost in the woods, for example, is an element in many fairy tales. Who among us has not heard or read some fairy tales by the Brothers Grimm where the little protagonists get lost in the woods and are forced to face, overcoming numerous trials and obstacles, evil witches, tremendous ogres and wild animals ready to threaten their very existence? Recall Hansel and Gretel, Tom Thumb, Little Red Riding Hood. Usually all the protagonists manage to come out of the woods, spiritually or materially enriched (treasure is not infrequently found) and transformed, they return to their origins.

V. Propp's work is also interesting for later developments. In his work "The Historical Roots of Fairy Tales" [5], he questions the origin of the emergence of folk tales, going so far as to speculate that there is a connection with the traditions and rituals of primitive communities. For example, in his studies, Propp finds that in ancient primitive communities, the forest was an elective site for initiation rites that marked the passage from childhood to adulthood. During these rites young boys were subjected to numerous trials that involved facing the adversities of the wild and natural environment around them. These trials included passing through the dark forest, losing the path, finding the shaman's hut, and finally returning to the village, no longer infants but adults. The fairy tale would thus be the way to re-enact, in narrative and symbolic form, the ancient rite of passage to adulthood for the young people of those lands.

The function of stories has also been much investigated in the field of psychoanalysis. Bruno Bettelheim, Austrian psychoanalyst famous for his studies on psychoanalysis applied to the developmental age, assigns a cathartic role to the fairy tale which is recognized as having an important-formative role for the child [6]. In the fairy tale, in the great novels of literature, in the theater and even in the cinema, contact with emotions narrated or represented by others, not implying direct involvement, allows one to acquire information concerning the possible ways of living and expressing various emotional experiences, thus facilitating the very possibility of processing them and making them useful in his life. It is as if, in doing so, the subject anticipates emotional experiences and ways to accept them.

This characteristic of narrative function accompanies us into adulthood as well. In the words of Eco [7], "walking through a narrative world has the same function as play does for a child. Children play with dolls, wooden horses or kites, to familiarize themselves with physical laws and the actions they will one day have to perform in earnest. Likewise, reading stories means playing a game through which we learn to make sense of the immensity of things that have happened and are happening and will happen in the real world. By reading novels we escape the anguish that grips us when we try to say something true about the real world. This is the therapeutic function of fiction and the reason why men, from the beginning of humanity, have been telling stories. Which then is the function of myths: to give form to the disorder of experience" (p. 107).

Long relegated to the world of literature and childhood, narratives have in more recent times become the subject of scholarly interest by different disciplines in the social field.

The same philosophy that, beginning with the conception of man of Cartesian memory (cogito ergo sum), had always denied to narrative the value attributed to rational thought has in recent decades approached the forms of discourse in everyday experience with increasing curiosity.

Beginning in the 1980s, a new awareness of the need for storytelling in human existence emerged. To the countless definitions used over time to qualify the true essence of human beings (homo sapiens, faber, economicus, etc.) Fisher first added that of *homo narrans* [8]. Fischer introduces the narrative paradigm to communication theory. That is, he argues that people are essentially storytellers and considers storytelling to be one of the oldest and most universal forms of communication among human beings, to the extent that the very decisions and actions we make would depend on approaching the social world according to a narrative logic.

In the 1990s, Jerome Bruner, a cognitivist psychologist, supported the idea that narrative is a tool for constructing meaning. In particular he analyzed how meanings are exchanged, communicated, and shared with others through storytelling. With Bruner comes the recognition of narrative as the main form of human knowledge.

According to him, human beings have an aptitude or predisposition to organize experience in narrative form because this would serve our need to give it specific meaning. Narrative is for Bruner a very important psychological mechanism, which we activate from childhood to fulfill a dual purpose simultaneously: on the one hand, to create knowledge of the world and, on the other hand, to experience it. Man is thus conceived as a storyteller (1990–1991), characterized by an innate need to reconstruct the events of one's life in the form of a narrative, whether written or oral. That is, narrative thinking would be aimed at understanding and related to the way individuals organize their experience.

The close link between storytelling and the ability to construct meaning becomes more evident in the reflections initiated by Weick on the process by which people give meaning to their collective experiences, termed sensemaking [9].

Weick was interested in studying the working mechanism of the meaning-making process. He argued that individuals are exposed to multifaceted and unordered streams of experience and through cognitive processes they are able to give order to these streams, bringing cause/effect relationships into play. The cognitive process initiated would generate maps, called causal maps, by which we can interpret our experiences, giving them meaning and logical order, and thus predispose our behavior. Central to the development of plausible meanings is the bracketing of cues from the environment, and the interpretation of those cues based on salient frames. Sensemaking is thus about connecting cues and frames to create an account of what is going on.

This continuous process of understanding events, called sensemaking, involves the ability to think in narrative terms [9]. According to Weick's theory, reality makes sense only through our cognitive processes and it has the sense we give it.

In storytelling, therefore, we attribute meaning to our history and our actions. Moreover, since the meaning of an experience can only be grasped retrospectively, storytelling represents the elective site of sensemaking, a cognitive process based on the continuous formulation and search for causal links between events [10].

This view of the sensemaking process has strong implications for "what" reality is. If reality only makes sense through our cognitive processes, this means that "external" reality is equivalent, for each subject, to the subject's reading of it. This does not mean that reality does not exist or that it is imagination or dream, but rather that reality is ambiguous and each person gives it "his" meaning.

Another interesting concept by Weick [11] is that of enactment and enacted environment that closely relates the meanings we make to the actions enacted in the external context: the individual has a subjective perception of reality, but more importantly, the individual constructs reality through such activation. The activated environment retroacts on the activating subjects, who then must behave accordingly with respect to the constructed reality.

Narrative activity, as a sensemaking process, assumes particular relevance in the face of events that seem to violate canonicity, that is, when something unexpected happens or something expected does not happen. In this situation of deviation from the expected pattern, storytelling offers the possibility of recomposing the broken order [12] and managing the unexpected. Sensemaking is the process of social construction that occurs when discrepant cues interrupt individuals' ongoing activity and involves the retrospective development of plausible meanings that rationalize what people are doing. The sensemaking process is in fact a continuous and retrospective process (we can only make sense of what has happened after something has happened), in which shocking episodes can also lead us to reconsider the meaning of previous experiences [9]. Probably if there were no exceptions, trauma difficulties there would be no stories either. In addition to bringing into play cognitive skills, useful in systematizing and ordinating reality, and symbolic skills (in transforming primary experience into a universe of meaning), storytelling is a creative process because it involves the ability to imagine alternatives [12] as there is never only one story to tell a situation.

The development of postmodern toward the end of the twentieth century [13, 14] introduces a relativist approach that denies the presence of universal truths and considers knowledge as fragmented. In this context skepticism toward the grand narratives of the past and the idea of a universal and stable truth prevails. Rather, the idea of relying on the narrative approach to generate new insights and offer stimuli for a deeper understanding of phenomena is spreading. But sensemaking becomes more complex. David Boje, a postmodern thinker in the field of management theory and organizational science, introduces the concept of homo fabulans by addressing the complexity of interpreting a fragmented, collective narrative. "Because some experiences do not have a linear sequence, they are difficult to tell as a 'coherent' story. Telling stories that lack coherence is contrary to modernity. However, in the postmodern condition, stories are more difficult to tell because experience itself is so fragmented and so full of chaos that fixing meaning or imagining coherence is fictitious" [15].

In such "turbulent contexts," according to the definition by Emery and Trist [16], more recently Maitlis and Sonenshein [17] suggest that the construction of shared meanings and emotion during crisis and change plays a significant role: in particular two actions associated with wisdom—updating and doubting—are essential to enable an adaptive rather than destructive role for shared meanings.

They remind us that sensemaking is not only an individual issue. In their reflections on social contexts characterized by crisis and change, Maitlis and Sonenshein [17] speak of a bottom-up process for social change. The sensemaking that is given to an issue of social significance in turn influences how individuals respond to it. This is particularly the case when a group of individuals together develop a shared understanding of the social significance of certain issues. Weick [18] identified such a case in the Workers' Defense Committee in Poland, whose collective sensemaking in the face of confining and coercive macrostructures led to micro-changes that resulted in widespread democratic social change.

5.2   The Semiotic Approach

We have seen that, in literature and social science, storytelling is related to a sensemaking function. But how is a story constructed? Through what tools do we analyze the meaning and meanings produced through it?

Semiotics is defined as the general science of signs, their production, transmission, and interpretation, or the ways in which something is communicated and signified, or an otherwise symbolic object is produced. The term semiotic was first used in the early 1900s to denote an autonomous discipline that had as its object the functioning of sign systems, whether natural or artificial.

It is used to analyze the contents and meanings of a text with the aim of understanding a particular phenomenon. An application of this discipline involves the analysis of communication materials and in general of various objects of analysis, defined as "texts." Semiotics is applied not only to verbal texts (a novel, a story, a newspaper article, etc.) but all objects and phenomena that convey articulated meaning.

In semiotics, the term "text" means any portion of reality that has meaning for someone, endowed with internal cohesion and coherence. This means that the term "text" has a broader meaning than how it is commonly understood in everyday language: written and spoken language are just some of the ways through which meanings are conveyed. Similarly, images and gestures can also be understood as expressions of a codified communicative language, based on signs, symbols, signals or other still elements that can be understood according to a shared meaning within certain contexts and social groups. In summary, text is defined as any product obtained through the use of an encoded communicative language, regardless of its media and expressive characteristics. Short stories can be considered texts, but not only. Even a painting can be considered a text, as can a poster or a commercial, a piece of music, and so on. Even natural conversations that circulate spontaneously in a given social context have over time become objects of study. A painting is a text (a visual text), but so are an advertisement, a piece of music, a design object, etc. [19].

Modern semiotics as an autonomous field of study began to take shape in the 20th century. Greimas is the best-known exponent of structural semiotics, one of the most popular and useful theories for semiotic text analysis. This is a theory that has its origins in linguistics and anthropology, beginning with the work that Propp had done on fairy tales and leading to the spread in the 1960s–1970s of the structural method in the analysis of narrative texts.

He developed his ideas between the 1960s and 1990s with the intention of arriving at a general model that can describe all forms of narrative. He developed his ideas between the 1960s and the 1990s with the intention of arriving at a general model capable of describing all forms of narrative or rather "narrativity." Narrativity is a fundamental concept for Greimas, upon which he developed his model for analyzing and decoding the deep structure of narrative texts and thus their meanings. Narrativity refers to the set of rules and elements that contribute to the composition of a narrative text. and that at the same time correspond to the way through which human beings interpret the world. The deep structure of narrative texts, including short stories, histories and narratives in general. This framework is based on the concept of "narrativity" and includes a number of key componentsOr rather, narrativity, because according to Greimas, narrativity is not only a feature of novellas and novels. It is rather a way through which human beings interpret the world [20].

His methodology is called structuralist because its focus is the organization of narrative according to which the text is understood as a system made up of surface and deep structures and multiple interconnected levels:

- at the deepest level there is the narrative skeleton, in which we find the fundamental values and meanings on which the text is based (e.g., the struggle between life and death, good and evil, etc.).
- on the surface there is everything we can see: the telling of the story, that is the words, colors, images, etc. The values that come from the deeper level here become the object of clashes, transformations, reversals.

One of the tools used by Greimas is the semiotic square, used to represent the fundamental relationships of meanings within a given semantic category. It is the most basic structure of the semantics of a text and establishes the most universal and general criteria of meaning, representing the general scheme of possible articulations in a given semantic category. That is, meaning values within the semiotic square are generated from their contrastive relations of differentiation, they always arise as opposite poles of a given semantic category by defining its particular variants by differentiation.[1]

Semiotic analysis is based on the analysis of different levels of the text and can proceed along two directions: from the surface to the deep or vice versa. The semiotic square leads to a kind of formal map that represents the functioning of a given semantic category through a differential geometric structure. It was this model that inspired the start of our work to analyze Social Dreaming matrices as texts and in particular the construction of Habitats as representations of mental maps of our inner world, as suggested by dreams.

References

1. Aristotele. Poetica. Milano: Bompiani; 2000.
2. Josselson R. Imagining the real: empathy, narrative, and the dialogic self. In: Josselson R, Lieblich A, editors. Interpreting experience: the narrative study of lives. London: Sage; 1995.
3. Spence D. Narrative truth and historical truth. New York: Norton; 1982.
4. Propp V. Morfologia della fiaba. Torino: Einaudi; 1928. p. 2000.
5. Propp V. Le radici storiche dei racconti di fate. Torino: Boringhieri; 1946. p. 1972.
6. Bettelheim B. Il mondo incantato: uso, importanza e significati psicoanalitici delle fiabe. Milano: Feltrinelli; 1977. p. 2001.
7. Eco U. Sei passeggiate nei boschi narrative. Milano: Bompiani; 1994.
8. Fisher WR. Human communication as narration: toward a philosophy of reason, value, and action. University of South Carolina Press; 1987.
9. Weick KE. Sensemaking in organizations. London: Sage; 1995.
10. Poggio B. Mi racconti una storia? Il metodo narrativo nelle scienze sociali. Roma: Carocci; 2004.
11. Weick KE. Enacted sensemaking in crisis situations. J Manag Stud. 1988;25:305–17.
12. Bruner J. Acts of meaning. Harvard University Press; 1990.
13. Foucalt M. L'archeologia del sapere. Milano: BUR; 1999.
14. Lyotard. La condizione postmoderna: rapporto sul sapere. Milano: Feltrinelli; 1979. p. 1981.
15. Boje DM. Narrative methods for organizational and communication research. London: Sage; 2001.
16. Emery FE, Trist EL. The causal texture of organizational environments. Hum Relat. 1965;18:1.
17. Maitlis S, Sonenshein S. Sensemaking in crisis and change: inspiration and insights from Weick. J Manag Stud. 2010;47:3.
18. Weick KE. Sensemaking as an organizational dimension of global change. In: Cooperider DL, Dutton JE, editors. Organizational dimensions of global change: no limits to cooperation. Sage; 1999. p. 39–56.
19. Marrone G. Corpi Sociali: Processi comunicativi e semiotica del testo. Torino: Einaudi; 2002.
20. Greimas A. Del senso. Milano: Bompiani; 1970. p. 2001.

---

[1] For example: the meaning Life (S1) is defined by its opposition to the concept of Death (S2) and vice versa. The presence of Life automatically recalls its opposite, Death. But not only that Greimas introduces, in addition to the two contrary elements (Life/Death), two other elements: the so-called contradictors (not S1 and not S2). In this sense Life is defined not only in relation to its opposite Death, but also to the contradictor, called non S1 (not Life). We can say that the opposite of Life, that is, Death (S2) is opposed to Life (S1), represents the other pole of that semantic category. The contradictory not S1, however, represents the negation of S1, it is "everything that is not Life."

Chapter 6
Social Dreaming Matrix as a Way to Build a Community of Intent: A Case History

6.1 EUNAMES, Medical Humanities and Narrative Medicine

EUNAMES, European Narrative Medicine Society, is the brainchild of the Italian Society of Narrative Medicine (SIMeN) and is a nonprofit group of health professionals, scholars and physicians, dedicated to researching and raising awareness of the issues of Narrative Medicine, Medical Humanities, and more generally Humanities for Health (disciplines that also include the relationship between the arts and therapies). The association is committed to improving the quality of health care systems at the national and European levels. The purpose of EUNAMES is to promote and strengthen dialogue about forms of Narrative Medicine and Health Humanities among health professionals who identify with this approach to health and wellness. EUNAMES recognizes that medicine, health care and social services are based on four principles: biological, psychological, social and spiritual or existential.

Its foundation is also favored by World Health Organization (WHO) as it provides an opportunity to build a network with people working on these issues, fostering exchange and discussion. It includes professionals coming from all over the world, researchers, academics, doctors, etc. Maria Giulia Marini is the founder and the current president.

By Narrative Based Medicine (NBM) we mean "the practice of medicine with the application of the skills of recognizing, including, understanding, and interpreting disease stories" [1].

The importance of storytelling in care settings is first recognized and formalized by Charon [2], a U.S. internist physician, who talks about Narrative Medicine (NM) by highlighting the benefit that disease stories have in patient care and the doctor–patient relationship. In the early 2000s, she founded the Program in Narrative Medicine at Columbia University in New York City. This program was one of the first to offer formal training in narrative medicine, bringing together the worlds of

© The Author(s), under exclusive license to Springer Nature Switzerland AG 2023
E. Pasini, C. Trimboli, *A Social Dreaming Experience at the Time of COVID 19*, New Paradigms in Healthcare, https://doi.org/10.1007/978-3-031-42498-4_6

medicine and the humanities. It aimed to teach healthcare professionals how to listen to and interpret patients' stories, recognizing that these narratives can provide valuable insights into their medical conditions and experiences. Awareness and attention to this field of study have been gradually growing in the medical community as more healthcare institutions and universities began incorporating narrative medicine principles into their training programs. It became clear that understanding the patient's narrative – their personal experiences, beliefs, and emotions – could improve the quality of healthcare by fostering better doctor-patient communication, empathy, and a deeper understanding of the patient's needs [3, 4].

Narrative medicine is part of the medical humanities an interdisciplinary field that explores the intersection of medicine, healthcare, and the humanities. It seeks to understand and improve the human experience of illness, healthcare delivery, and the practice of medicine through the lens of literature, art, philosophy, ethics, history, and other humanities disciplines. The philosophical and social science fields are those in which reflections on narrative originated and have become increasingly relevant over time. Medical humanities use interdisciplinary research to explore experiences of health and illness, often focusing on subjective, hidden, or invisible experience. But more broadly we may say that the roots of Narrative Medicine can be found in art whenever through figurative and literary works the theme of health and illness has been given space. In the words of Maria Giulia Marini [5, 6], one of the most authoritative voices of Narrative Medicine in Italy, "we can say that true narrative medicine was born when it stopped being a narrated novel [5]."

In brief, Narrative Medicine began to shape as a field of studies because of the need to humanize medical practice, emphasizing the importance of understanding and incorporating the narratives of patients and healthcare providers into medical care. NM grew out of a critical approach to the Evidence-Based Medicine (EBM) model that had been introduced in the 1970s in response to the need for standardization in clinical research methodology and which, over time, had become the elective reference point in medical practice. In fact, over time, an awareness developed of the need to integrate this approach to a different framework for health care, more aimed at humanizing care. The goal of MN is to recover a holistic view of the patient and the disease [1].

In Europe, NM developed from a publication by B. Hurwitz and T. Greenhalgh in the British Medical Journal [7] that voiced criticism of evidence-based medicine (EBM). In fact, over time, a conscientiousness had emerged that it was not possible to apply comprehensive medicine to the individual case but that it was necessary to gather the patient's history beyond the history, to listen to the person beyond the patient. Only in this way it is possible in medical practice to contextualize objective signs and symptoms of illness with respect to the patient's world (values, places, relationships), recovering a look, in the approach to care, that is more complex and more integrated.

NM takes the form of an approach that broadens the traditional scientific vision, adding a more enlarged and "humanized" look at the patient, aware of the importance that, in the care relationship, has the experiences and the very way of telling one's disease history. In this new framework, instead of "disease," which expresses an organic view of pathology, considered a biological alteration and dysfunction, the term "illness" is preferred, which instead encompasses the experience brought by the person about his or her illness, his or her narrative [8].

In NM, the call for medical and nursing professionals is to recover a humanistic view of care, this made possible through the use of a narrative approach, which allows for the recovery of broader meanings attributed to health and illness. Today, the increasing attention to the narrative strand affirms the idea that it is inherent in stories to acquire better psychological well-being.

6.2 The Experience of Social Dreaming in EUNAMES

In the spring of 2021 Maria Giulia Marini contacted us to ask us to implement for the EUNAMES group a Social Dreaming course similar to the one she had taken part in during the lockdown. She had participated in the Social Dream Matrices experience we conducted during the pandemic in 2020 and was so positively impressed by it that she wanted to repeat it within EUNAMES, of which she was president moved by the idea that it could be an important moment of expressiveness, after the pandemic, for the members of the group. She had read Gordon Lawrence's book and knew of his use of Social Dreaming in organizations during his experiences at the Tavistock Institute in London.[1]

The need to apply this method to the EUNAMES group as well stemmed from the need to redefine the Community's charter of values that existed at that time and had been the result of desk-based, rational, and standardized work. Rather, there was a need to tap into the Community's value assets in a deeper and more authentically expressive way, in order to use it as a means of internal communication and deep collective identification. In this sense, Maria Giulia felt that Social Dreaming could be a valuable tool.

The aim was allowing to make connections and sharing dreams in order to create together new meanings, searching for less obvious pillars through social dreaming session among the members of EUNAMES.

At the time SD began the declared pillars of EUNAMES were:

- Plurality of approaches
- Inclusivity
- Multidisciplinary
- Open to every country also outside Europe
- Community of practice

It was a desk-written charter of values that even though they were agreeable and "politically correct" turned out to be rather standardized. Rather, it was intended, through Social Dreaming, to find a way more authentically connected to the deep identity of EUNAMES.

---

[1] Dr. Lawrence saw the possibility of dreaming socially, not about "me" but about the human condition. In the spring of 1982, with psychoanalyst Patricia Daniels, a colleague, he began holding weekly "Social Dreaming Sessions" at the Tavistock, called A Project in Social Dreaming and Creativity and subsequently held Social Dreaming conferences in London, Birmingham, and Ireland. Social Dreaming has flourished in Israel, Sweden, Germany, France, Italy, the USA, Ireland, Finland, Rwanda, South Africa, Holland, Denmark, Australia, and India. Social Dreaming is now the subject of substantial academic study. It has been used to surface creativity, tackle management issues, understand social issues in disparate groups, surface unconscious issues at conferences, and foster innovation in for-profit, nonprofit, government, education, political, and other organizations.

Participants were about ten persons, involved in the sessions. It was a very international group, this was particularly interesting for us to see how and how much the pandemic had been able to generate connections, resonances, similarities in the collective imagination. Participants were mostly from Europe (UK, Greece, Germany, Ireland, Portugal, Italy, Spain) and more marginally also from Africa (UAE) and South America (Mexico). The sessions were conducted in English.

We explained that the SD was a place for sharing and trying to investigate what was happening at the level of the unconscious, which means dreams, feelings, etc. We tried to reassure that the sharing would have allowed to understand not something regarding just the singular individuals, but something that would have given new meanings in what was happening to them. We would have tried to expand the connections of the people in the group through the dreams. We carried out a Social Dreaming Matrix journey based on 3 online meetings, conducted on a monthly basis, between February and April 2021. The historical moment was that of the second phase of the pandemic, marked by the start of vaccination. The meetings were carried out in the manner and timing of the experience carried out the year before during the lockdown in Italy. Each session lasted 2 hours, one hour was devoted to the Dream Matrix, 45' to the Reflection Group. Each Matrix was followed by a staff meeting. The group of the participants was formed on a voluntary base, as a dreamlike exploration of the imagery of the EUNAMES group at that time. The group consisted of physicians and Narrative Medicine scholars. The staff was composed by the host of the Matrix and one co-host helping for the operative aspects. The 3 SDMs were held online in a Zoom platform. Participants were asked to freely and spontaneously share their dreams, with no self-presentations and interpretations. At the end of the experience a final meeting was held, on May 2021 to present and discuss the suggestions of the landscape of dreams developed by the collection of images of the staff.

Below we briefly present the work done in the Matrices and the results that emerged. After each Social Dreaming session, we worked on collecting the dreams and transposing them into images in order to analyze the meanings and symbols that emerged. Again at the end of each matrix we made a map, which we shared with group members and used to activate new reflections, links, and connections.

Our task was to bring to the group's attention the main themes and areas of meaning emerging from the dreams, to develop maps of the imaginary the oneiric, and to foster, through sharing and reflection, the participants' expressiveness.

The **first matrix** developed around a dual opposition: Individual versus Collective, then Mind versus Body. The dreams spoke of gifts given, images and situations related to spirituality, deaths, and funerals. The evoked spirituality was contrasted with other images where a sensoriality of bright colors, corporeality, Arabian markets, and walks in unfamiliar places stood out. There was also a reference to ancestral figures, ancestors (especially female figures), and a certain nostalgia for origins. These were contrasted with images of single furniture, accompanied by a sense of disorientation and loss.

The **second matrix** brought out two contrasts: between desire for movement and stationary, between appeasement and authenticity. In the dreams masks were removed, there was a sense of fear, disorientation in unfamiliar places, the idea of having to start over. There were frequent scenes of travel and discovery, a recurring theme being the exploration of faraway places where there was music, well-being, bright colors, and a widespread sense of freedom. Alternating with these scenes were more intimate settings, images of old childhood photographs and family lunches, familiar places that evoked nostalgia for the old days.

In the **third matrix** the dreamlike imagery told developed along the juxtaposition of obedience versus breaking the rules, light versus night landscapes. The dreams recalled the experience of swimming in the sea, among polluted water, dark own side, and big mountain to climb. There was the search for healthy water. Blindfolded guesses raised the paradox of being blind and the question: who is blind?

The meanings identified, based on the oppositions that emerged during the matrices, were shared at the end of the course with the participants. This work was then the subject of an internal group reflection that led to the definition of a new EUNAMES values charter.

The final work was considered successful by Maria Giulia Marini: "It gave depth and meaning to stated values and expressed new values." It finalized certain values that could never have been defined by relying on rational thinking alone and allowed for a better declination and deepening of the meaning of some of the starting values.

Through work with SD matrices, EUNAMES has come to define these values, shown below with a brief description by keywords:

- The association of interest
- Restorative justice
- Getting lost
- Spiritual and grounded
- Appraisal of every kind of knowledge
- From ancestors to next generations

The presentation of values took place at the EUNAMES European Congress, held in Porto in May 2022. These are inspirational values of EUNAMES that created excitement and interest in some, especially among younger people, but at the same time also some skepticism from those who labeled the method used unorthodox for a scientific community.

Nevertheless the work done served to get to know each other better created a space where everyone told their own "truths" through dreams and strengthen the group's sense of identity.

> Many of us teach, we have academic roles...people's frailties and insecurities came out, the sense of being lost...this created humanity...We got to know each other better, we threw down the mask...it also served me a lot as a guiding compass, on how to manage the group...

Some participants spontaneously sent feedback immediately after the experience, communicating to us satisfaction and some gratitude for the application of the method. Others were contacted after a while and through an open-ended questionnaire sent us a brief comment on the experience.

None of them was familiar with the SD methodology before their experience together.

The initial reaction to Maria Giulia Marini's invitation to participate was full of ambivalence: the very idea of being able to share dreams within a social space in total openness and freedom at the same time created curiosity and interest as well as aroused apprehension because it involved sharing with other people the contents of one's dreams that could be intimate and personal.

> The concept itself immediately caught my attention, considering the dire times we are living in and through: the idea of dreams entering the social space - infusing it with endless possibilities, openness, liminality, freedom - is not just welcomed, it is fundamental.
> The experience of a Social Dreaming matrix was an extraordinary one, as it demanded begin totally open in front of a group of strangers.

The matrices were experienced as a unique experience, with a particular climate they truly appreciated: the dimension of confidentiality, even with people never seen before, the sense of community, the deep respect for other people's experience.

> The experience of a Social Dreaming matrix was an extraordinary one, as it demanded begin totally open in front of a group of strangers.
> I enjoyed the intimacy of the souls (although these are people I have never met in person and the sessions were via the internet), the sincerity of the participants and the confidence that what is said is confidential within the group. I think that the common scientific backgrounds and common scientific interests of the participants, the mature age and the mutual respect contributed to these.
> The sense of enthusiasm for experiencing something completely new but at the same time something very familiar.

Beyond the aspects of climate generated in the group, what was striking was the content of the matrices: through the meetings an awareness of common elements that united, levels of interconnectedness between people took hold. It also increased the level of knowledge that was less superficial and more intimate, deep, facilitated by a more informal and free conversation, freed from the role positions one had within the group. Within the matrix were people, with their human frailties; the "masks" dictated by hierarchical positions had fallen away.

It struck the commonality of themes, of recurring symbols, which turned out to strengthen a reassuring bond among the participants.

> I was surprised by the fact that, with the passing of time, a bond developed between the participants in the meetings which only they understood.
> During the first meeting I attended, I felt like I was witnessing a particular kind of knowledge being created, one that is encompassing, lively, and fluid, that follows a non-hierarchical approach to episteme, that is bent on equality, relationality and interdependence. This is the kind of knowledge that is informed by theory and practice, but which comes from a deeper place: necessity. Is is indeed a necessary knowledge, vital not only to the (often challenging) dialogue between Health and Humanities, but also to our human existence, stifled as it is today by fear and uncertainty.
> I was amazingly surprised by the common matrices among the participants.
> People living thousands of kilometers far …. They were experiences same fears, same sense of loss, same uncertainty. This gave to me the real sense of a Universal Soul that is connecting all people in the world. This "Sympathy" stream is flowing through people with even more strength in case of common universal catastrophes (like the pandemic, currently the war etc). I was surprised (and got a sense of comfort in the same time) by the common presence of Ancestors/Family in our Dreams. This is just confirming "We are our own Stories" and in difficult times, our own Story comes somehow overpowering our daily life in order to give us clues and paths to follow. And this is somehow so reassuring!

Participation had also generated in some a greater production of night dreams during the period of the meetings and greater attention to their emotional sphere.

> I dreamed more during the weeks it took place and remembered my dreams more.
>   My desire to be concentrated on my dreams in that period (I started writing my dreams in the morning paying attention to my emotions and feelings)

With respect to the pandemic, the opportunity to explore and discover the meeting points of shared imagery was appreciated.

> The most valuable thing was the opportunity to experience the pandemic together. I think this experience has left me with a deeper perception of the pandemic.

Nevertheless, the methodology, which involved personal exposure and a certain repetitiveness, created some resistance that led some of the participants to abandon the final session.

> I had written down the dream that I had seen after participating to a session and considered very important, but in the last moment I could not bring myself to open the computer, pretended -also to myself-that I was too busy. Now I have regretted this.

What remains, in the balance of the experience, is the idea of having done something of value and of having strengthened the group's collective bond and identity through dreams. And the desire to want to follow up on the experience.

> I thought it was an effective way of helping a group to bond and creating intimacy and trust.
>   I learnt dreams are able to create intimate Connection among people and this is so reassuring and fascinating!
>   A sense of friendliness and trust within the group. Greater respect for community and openness to new things. An impression that we all shared similar preoccupations, particularly around Covid.
>   I valued it mainly as a way of helping to group to become more cohesive in its identity. I regretted that I wasn't able to attend all the sessions.
>   Now is the time to dream as a way to expand and connect, which reminds me here of Adrienne Rich's understanding of poetry as being moved by "the drive / to connect. The dream of a common language" ("Origins and History of Consciousness"). I believe Social Dreaming is guided by a similar willingness to connect, based on a common language between "I" and "other," between Health and Humanities, Art and Science.
>   I didn't like that after Social dreaming experience was over , I stopped writing my dreams in the morning ;-(
> The desire to participate more. I have tried to find worthy practices in Greece, but without success so far.

6.3   Conclusions

The tool of Social Dreaming demonstrated some effectiveness in achieving the purpose. The sharing of dreams in an extended context became an opportunity for deep expressiveness, allowed to experience on oneself experiences of hopelessness, fragility that are inherent in the topics covered by medical humanities and narrative medicine. It is possible to say that it created a space for caring for the soul of the group.

Certainly experience also highlights the light and dark of the application of Social Dreaming in organizational contexts. It must be kept in mind that some people have a mindset that prefers methodologies that bring numerical evidence and give less credence to forms of knowledge based on other research paradigms.

In conclusion, some useful suggestions for conducting future interventions can be drawn from this experience.

Undoubtedly one of the strengths highlighted is the ability to activate and "cultivate" symbolic thinking: through work in the matrix, multiplicities of ideas and images emerge, in a freer and more facilitating setting than in more formalized and institutionalized meeting moments.

At the same time, there are some weaknesses that need to be aware of. Personal resistance may emerge, during the matrix, due to fear of exposing oneself and showing "shadow" sides to other participants. More introverted personality traits may find it more difficult to approach the methodology than those who are more extroverted, more naturally willing to open up to others. This brings to mind the importance of the role of the SD host, where working with a group, as a facilitator to create a trusting, nonevaluative environment in which everyone can feel free to "throw down the mask."

Another resistance may come from a certain skepticism within the scientific community in recognizing the value of a dream-based methodology, which can easily be confused with new age, spiritual and alternative theories to the mainstream, with little theoretical foundation. This suggests that more dissemination and awareness of the great work done on Social Dreaming at the Tavistock by Gordon Lawrence, the methodology's founder, and subsequent developments, areas of application and achievements would be needed. In general, giving more prominence to scientific publications on dreaming could help overcome skepticism. Another useful thing might be to combine the methodology with fact-checking actions, to give evidence through quantitative surveys before or after the experience the added value, through measurable variables (e.g., tests of perceived stress) that SD can bring on the well-being of those taking part.

References

1. Marini MG. Languages of care in narrative medicine. Words, space and time in the healthcare ecosystem. London: Springer; 2019.
2. Charon R. Narrative medicine: form, function and ethics. Ann Intern Med. 2001;134:83–7.
3. Charon R. Narrative and medicine. NEJM. 2004;350:862.
4. Charon R. Narrative medicine. Honoring the stories of illness. New York: Oxford University, Press; 2006.
5. Marini MG. La Medicina narrativa nei luoghi di formazione e di cura. Milano: Edi Ermes; 2010.
6. Marini MG. Narrative medicine: bridging the gap between evidence-based care and medical humanities. London: Springer; 2016.
7. Greenhalgh T, Hurwitz B. Narrative based medicine: why study narrative? BMJ. 1999;318:48–50.
8. Kleinman A. The illness narratives: suffering, healing, and the human condition. Basic Books; 1988.

Chapter 7
A Tentative Conclusion: Dream Journeys as a Way towards a Collective Becoming

7.1 Living in the Meantime: The Moments of Passage in Life

A time, ours, which like others of the past, but much more radically, is characterised as a time of no longer and not yet, in which something still seems to exist, remains pending but weighs on and in everyone's lives, and something is beginning or has already begun but one finds it hard to recognize it and is afraid to name it. A 'meantime' with all the opportunities and dangers it contains.

    Mapelli, B., [1], Nuove intimità. Strategie affettive e comunitarie nel pluralismo contemporaneo (New Intimacies. Affective and community strategies in contemporary pluralism)

We live in difficult times, in which the anxieties and fears unleashed over the past 2 years by the pandemic are amplified today by the specter of a global war.

At times like these it is no longer possible to imagine a future without questioning ourselves and the fragile balance on which global society stands.

Three years after the pandemic, which represented a great divide in the Italian society and the world, what remains of that traumatic experience? What reflections? What is the lesson we can take from it?

It is widely believed that the pandemic represented a moment of crisis, an accelerator of change that altered our lives and our way of thinking. But it is not the only one. According to a recent article published in British economic media, the term "polycrisis" well defines the contemporary world, characterized by many major crises: in addition to the health crisis, in fact, the economic, climate, and political crises amplify the already widespread uncertainties about the future, which in the absence of certain points of reference exacerbate fears, disorientation, liability.

The need for a restart after COVID set in motion lot of energies, both positive and negative, sign of a common feeling that the pandemic bore many fruits, engendering expectations of a real change and desires to look to the future with new eyes.

E. Pasini, C. Trimboli, *A Social Dreaming Experience at the Time of COVID 19*, New Paradigms in Healthcare, https://doi.org/10.1007/978-3-031-42498-4_7

At the same time, however, a widespread concern that the expected change is not a given enhanced the experience of the disconnection between expectations and reality, between the inner and the outer world, making us feel uneasy and unprepared to face the change.

The image of "the bud blooming from the rubble" that emerged from the Italian Listening Post held in January 2023 is a good example to highlight important aspects of the contrasts we experience today.

The feeling shared by all the participants to the Listening Post was that the past few years of the pandemic were characterized by mixed feelings. On the one hand, energy and desire for a renewal at the end of the health emergency after the COVID pandemic; on the other hand, the deep feeling of living in a moment of transition, in which it is difficult to make sense of what is happening because of the disconnect between the expectations for change that we had harbored for 2 years and the return to a normalcy with which we are not satisfied. Faced with such contrasts, the prevailing emotions are expectation, depression, confusion, and hope. The image of "letting the bud inside you blossom", emerged from the January 2023 Listening Post session), sounds like a wish that holds opposite meanings: on the one side embodies a potential for growth, but on the other side represents the tendency to take refuge in oneself, an introspective movement to seek protection from a harsh reality and to escape anxiety. The bud may represent the hope that flowers blossom amid the rubble, but it is also fatigue, a bun to cling to in order to counter fear. The inner journey of the past 2 years of pandemic may have given us a better awareness of our inner feelings and emotions, but now it is time to come to terms with a reality that no longer corresponds to the expectations.

In the social sphere in fact the small signs of openness and recognition fail to counteract a stalemate at work, and companies and institutions seem unable to correspond to the many requests of organizational change.

The economic and social crisis and the war exacerbate aggression, violence, fragmentation, and the feeling of living a highly regressive moment in the social environment enhances conflicts, aggression, frustration, sense of powerlessness. The world seems to be drifting and we do not feel equal to the situation, unable to act effectively in the face of disaster.

If the COVID has made us more aware on an inner level, it has also increased our fears, and the temptation to take refuge in our inner world, to call ourselves out of the game. We seek inner balance and individual growth, we embrace meditation and mindfulness. But in the long run, might these not just be defenses against a more responsible engagement in the world? Is it possible to combat the social media superficial cacophony taking refuge in one's inner world? Have we really come out of the pandemic "bubble," or are we still trapped in a prison made of inner alibis?

The misalignment between major social issues (war, pandemic, climate crisis) and individual behaviors has reached a high level of risk that can no longer be reconciled. Face to an increasingly threatening social environment, states and governments react in a disorganized, paranoid, meaningless way.

Constantly oscillating between an individual sense of "autistic isolation" on the one side, and a constant drive to enact a "compulsive sociability" on the other side, we have lost a sense of "WE" and have not even the vaguest idea of what could be done to restore a new one. Yet, we cultivate the hope that flowers can be born from rubble; and if it is true that digging the rubble flowers may blossom from earth, everyone is now called upon to play their own responsibility. If in a moment of transition and deep uncertainty we feel the collective dimension of WE is far from coming, we should at least ask ourselves why it's missed so badly, and why should be essential to cultivate it today?

We have already pointed out that the so called "moments of passage", or transitional stages of life, accompany us throughout from when we are born to when we die, and without them there could be no healthy development.

People' s lives are made up of many different phases: we grow up from childhood to adulthood; we fall in love, marry, and separate; we go through births and deaths of our loved ones; we move from different countries, change jobs, meet new people, and leave others behind. The complexity of the contemporary age is such that the statement that "transits never end" applies even more today [2, p. 9].

In the absence of a clear and defined vision of the future, our contemporary time takes the form of a "meantime," to quote Barbara Mapelli [1]. In the meantime that is our life today, we live "as if" we were passing through a middle ground, suspended between a past that is no longer there and a future that has not yet taken full shape.

Personal biographies are subject today to constant changes, transitions, misplacements, and reinventions that take the form of journeys without safe landings. Our lives are similar to the *Interrupted Paths* spoken by the philosopher Martin Heidegger [3], in comparison to the walks of the philosopher in the forests near home, because just as wandering around in the forest one could easily lose the main path, so human thought should not set itself a definitive goal, but proceed by constant detours, wandering along impervious paths.

Traditional cultures of the past had initiation rituals that enabled people to cope with the most important transitional moments of life, like i.e. changements of age, gender, status. These institutional containers supported individuals in crossing the middle ground between the no longer and the not-yet, which thus became a space of exploration and discovery. Unlike in the past, however, all these stages of life are today mostly experienced in solitude, often perceived as existential crisis bringing anxiety and uncertainty about the future and questioning one's identity, which requires a radical change of attitudes and behaviors.

Today the multiplication and acceleration of moments of transition are individual experiences that occur in the absence of collective containers, increasing the sense of isolation and the risk of being locked inside an "autistic bubble."

Today, it is no longer possible to imagine a future without questioning ourselves and the fragile balance on which global society rests. In order to re-imagine a future together, it is essential to adopt a position of listening to others and a view of the world open to confrontation and differences.

> We lack today individual and collective settings as containers to provide space for new points of view to grow. Indeed, the fluid complexity of the 'meantime' requires an active and collaborative attitude that can give direction to the ongoing transformations [2, p. 19].

Recovering a ritualized dimension of moments of transition contributes to creating transitional spaces as collective moments of re-elaboration that sustain the I in the face of the speed and quantity of external changes.

The pandemic has increased loneliness and isolation but it has also heightened our awareness of how important the collective dimension is for linking individual and social change; at the same time, it has made us realize the urgency of recovering a collective dimension to bring transformative thinking to life.

At the beginning of 2020, the pandemic was the impetus for us to look for a new way of dealing with difficult transitional moments in life, and dreams have "enlightened" us along the way. We believe that such "moments of transition" are opportunities to better understand the changes taking place within and around us and to increase the awareness of the inner potential that can lead to surprising new discoveries.

We are probably experiencing the greatest revolution in human history, in terms of the intensity and rapidity of the changes taking place that affect the living, environmental, working, economic, and social contexts in which we live. Looking at what the pandemic has been for the outside world, it is possible to say that it has probably played the role of an accelerator of something that was already in the air but had not yet fully manifested itself, placing us today in front of absolutely new scenarios, with characteristics of high speed, unpredictability, and impact of change, driven by a technological change that opens up hybrid worlds, with a strong contamination between real and digital [4].

How to survive in this new context characterized by such rapid and profound changes and to cope with the challenges, including the existential ones, that it poses?

The ESCO18 classification confirms the central importance of activating and developing the so-called transversal skills, which can enable to play an active and conscious role in the processes of continuous change to which we are subjected. These are skills that are not learnt through classic training methods but require the activation of an experiential and reflective training model, according to the lifelong learning model.

The pandemic allowed us to set out on a journey, to discover our inner selves, our loneliness, our frailties, but also to bring to light the inner resources we can activate.

In this discovery we found ourselves connected to others. Recalling the words of Borgna [5], an Italian psychiatrist, *it was like an indispensable journey not only to the knowledge of what we are and of what others are, because no one knows himself until he explores his loneliness through the eyes of others.*

7.2   The Dream Journeys and the Power of Imagination

We have to get better at believing the impossible! (Kevin Kelly, founder of the Wired magazine)
Beneath the pavement endless beaches! (Slogan of the May '68 French movement)

Few years ago, at the mid of the 1990s and the beginning of the new millennium, the "world wide web" of the origins heralded a web culture based on concepts such as open source, peer to peer, social networks; a language of "hope and openness" that seemed to anticipate the expectation, shared by many, that a new era was about to come. The main protagonists of the so-called new economy imagined a world founded on the free circulation of ideas, open flexible communities, decentralized networks, leaderless organizations. Inspired by principles such as free participation, widespread democracy, respect for differences, the flurry of optimism that accompanied the new global world suggested that the totalitarian ideologies of the nineteenth century could finally be discarded as distant memories.

In the last decade, however, the many dramatic changes in the global context have revived the ghosts of the past, whose voice resounds loud and clear today. Wars and battles of conquest, nationalisms, totalitarianisms, divisions between the states, walls and barriers at the borders, migrations, mass exoduses, pandemics have definitely weakened the pioneering spirit, and the global utopia of a perfectly regulated world has been replaced with a myriad of dystopian worlds in perennial fight one another. Something in the most recent years has got out of control, the Western faith in an unlimited progress has vanished, the belief in a better world has turned into a nightmare. The idea of the future as a linear progression of continuous improvements that, thanks to technological and scientific development, enhances the living standards of many, which guided the western world for centuries, sounds now problematic, vague, threatening. In such an unpredictable social context individual destinies and multiple identities play a prominent role in retrieving the ghosts of the past, and social media emphasize the fracture between a subject tenaciously anchored to its individuality and a collective orphaned of common values.

Today, we feel we are living in a "dystopian world," in which the dark powers of the collective unconscious dominate unleashed and unacknowledged, and the capacity to symbolize and explore new meanings is constantly undermined by an inflation of mindless representations of reality. We are increasingly unable to connect conscious and unconscious contents, giving space to those creative hidden sides of the unconscious that could open access to an expanded consciousness of the world.

To build a better future, however, we should cultivate the ability to nurture an "expectation of the extraordinary" that fuels imagination. To plan the future, we must first be able to imagine it; and what we have lost today, and need more than anything else, is to regain confidence in the power of imagination.

J.K. Rowlings, the creator of Harry Potter, called imagination the ability to share with others what we consider essential. A capacity, Rowlings says,

> … that requires taking action, because it's only thanks to the courage of taking risks and making mistakes and the ability to learn from one's frailties that we can distinguish what is truly essential from what is not; and therefore, there is no need for magic to transform the world if you have the gift of imagination. (Rowlings J.K., On Failure and Imagination, speech for the Harvard University Academic year, June 2008)

Would it then be possible to look at the many phenomena of unpredictable change that are constantly before our eyes, and that worry us so much, not only as manifestations of an uncontrolled dynamic between dark forces, but rather as opportunities for new discoveries, possibilities to shed light on parts of the reality that we can no longer understand? Quoting a famous metaphor, if the black swans outnumber today the white ones, is not it a sign that something is happening at a deeper level, that requires full attention? We have an enormous need to nurture imagination, to search for scraps of meaning, to disseminate utopias, thus giving space to the imaginative function of the psyche. These are the dimensions that deserve to be explored today in order to recover a sense of "us" and new forms of coexistence in which the past is not a burden to get rid of but an opportunity to imagine a better possible future together. We need to recover a sense of community, to look at the bonds that unite us in an "invisible network of correspondences," which enhances our sense of belonging and makes us feel we are not living in isolation. Similar to the notion of "ubuntu" that inspired Nelson Mandela and Archbishop Desmond Tutu's South African Reconciliation Committee:

> God has given us a great gift, ubuntu… Ubuntu says I am human only because you are human… I need other persons to become a person myself… We don't come fully formed into the world. We learn how to think, how to walk, how to speak, how to behave, indeed how to be human from other human beings. We need other human beings in order to be human. We are made for togetherness, we are made for family, for fellowship, to exist in a tender network of interdependence. ('God is not a Christian'—An interview with Archbishop Emeritus Desmond Tutu in Cape Town, South Africa by Christian Egge)

Our hyper-connected digital world provides many contents, but few containers for the co-creation of common experiences. Working on dreams, we argue, allows that the process of connection between conscious and unconscious contents that Jung called the "transcendent function," which that is so necessary to overcome a situation of collective trauma.

We have highlighted before how the Dream Journey of the 4 Social Dreaming Matrices we undertook with other fellow travelers in the early days of the pandemic was the result of an intuition rather than a plan. Soon, however, we realized that, through dreams, the experience had turned into a journey of self-awareness and self-discovery of internal resources we did not know we had.

Those discoveries guided us through the transition from a kind of "magical thinking"—a kind of autistic anti-thinking based on self-reclosure, denial of reality and fantasies of omnipotence that preclude the possibility of a real confrontation with the other—to a "transformative thinking," that nurtures creativity, imagination, individual responsibility, in a confrontation with the unconscious in which seeing one's own fears reflected in the eyes of the other allows a change of perspective and the building of mutual bonds.

To highlight the discoveries and learnings made in each of the 4 stages of the journey, we now propose to use the metaphor of the "4 Treasure Island Archipelago," where each island corresponds to the emotional landscape explored in the 4 Social Dreaming Matrices. In the four stages of our dream journey we landed on four different islands. In each one of them we have been confronted with fears, anxieties, different emotions, that challenged our inner balance. But in each one of them we also found an unexpected treasure of inner resources, a precious source of

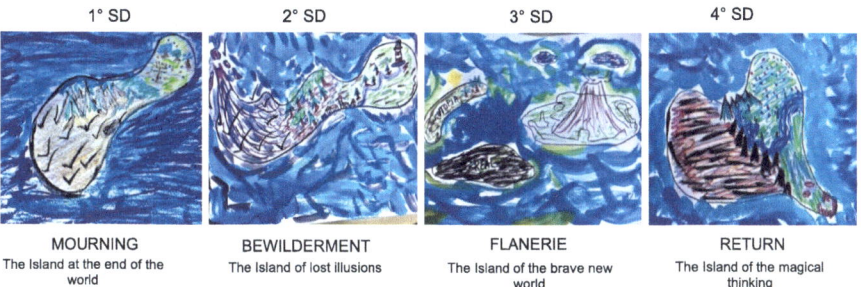

Fig. 7.1   The dreams journey. (*Images by Elisabetta Pasini*)

learning pointing the way to a possible becoming. We now therefore suggest to explore together the 4 islands as a metaphor of an "archipelago of conflicting emotions," where each one of them represents an emotional landscape that allows one to pause in uncertainty, contain anxieties and fears, discover inner personal resources.

We believe in fact that Dream Journey is a fundamental tool today to combine the evocative power of dreams with the need to find new reference points, new maps in order to move more easily in the new territory that is emerging. Our proposal is at the same time the way to find a safe and secure space to process together with others a collective trauma, or, more simply, a tool to deepen, together with other fellow travelers, the need to understand, through dreams, where we are heading to, bringing together introspective capacity and common feeling, and nourishing the desire for a different way of sociality, different forms of intimacy.

The journey through the four islands - depicted in Fig. 7.1–7.5 - is therefore not only the final stage of the adventure. It aims to be, above all, a proposal for a safe and secure container that, in times of turbulence and collective crisis, is essential to process disruptive changes, enhancing the social understanding for a collective becoming (Fig. 7.1).

7.3   The Treasure at the End of the Story: Learnings from the Dream Journey

7.3.1   The Island at the End of the World

See Fig. 7.2.

The first Social Dreaming Matrix on March 17 2020 confronted us with the end of a way of life. We had to endure the pain of loss, trying to figure out how to come to terms with the unexpected that suddenly had wiped out all that was familiar, taken for granted, and made our lives safe and secure.

The world we knew had suddenly dissolved, leaving behind a sense of loss for the end of a way of living and all its certainties, a void that was as inevitable as fate.

Fig. 7.2 SDM 1:
Mourning

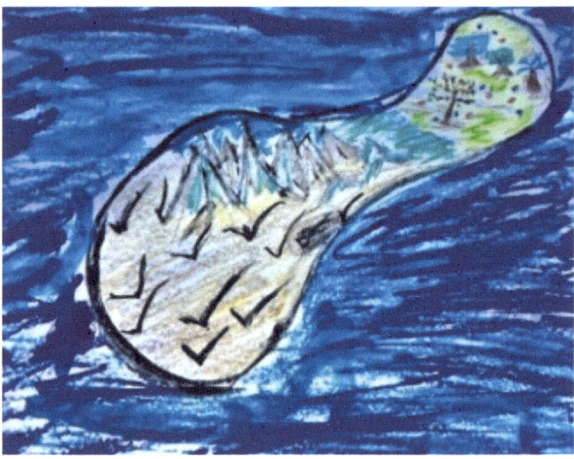

The first island we encountered along the way was therefore the "Island at the End of the World." All the destructive emotions related to loss—sadness, despair, loneliness, fear, betrayal—reinforced the sudden discovery of how fragile, endangered, exposed, and vulnerable we were. Moreover, we felt we were alone with our fears, because all the social occasions that gave a rhythm to our lives - school, work, entertainment, sport, friendship - had suddenly disappeared, leaving behind only a distorted, virtual image of itself.

The mourning process always requires "letting go" of something, and the exploration of the first island was, at first, a way of dealing with grief, learning how to get rid of some of the ghosts that haunted us. Along the way, however, we slowly understood how to deal with frailties and how to test our strengths. We had to choose what to keep and what to leave behind, and making choices we realized that was up to us to decide how heavy our baggage should be.

The most important discovery we made in the first island was therefore that getting rid of the ballast of the past to get to the essentials is not a job one can do alone. The first discovery was how much we needed a common space for sharing, a space in which is possible seeing and being seen by others, acknowledging ones strengths and weaknesses, as well as ones defenses and resources.

The learning of the first island was to realize that a traumatic experience could also be a valuable opportunity for renewal. When shared with others, instead of a source of suffering in isolation the dread of an inescapable individual fate, a collective trauma it may be a valuable opportunity for a change of perspective, from the isolation of the I to the collective becoming of the WE.

Emotions	Resources
• Sadness	• Regret
• Uncertainty	• Fragility
• Loneliness	• Letting go
• Betrayal	• Need for community

7.3.2   The Island of Lost Illusions

See Fig. 7.3.

In the second SDM, the second step of the journey brought us to the Island of the Lost Illusions, in which the shadows became thicker, more threatening and dangerous than ever, but also more concrete.

In the second island, we realized that, to find a new balance, we have to endure the thrill of imbalance. For it is only when it seems that all is lost that we may find the unexpected resources that allow a sudden leap, a flick of the wrist, an instinctive reaction.

Overwhelmed by a danger against which we felt powerless we had lost all capacity to react, fear had turned into panic. But when all hope seems lost, when all the coping strategies seem useless and futile, when all other possibilities have faded away, a new vital, primitive, instinctive energy comes to the rescue as an unexpected resource.

It is in these moments that we realize we can rely on improvisation, the power of the instinctive gesture, on that flicker of intuition that helps to distinguish real dangers from imaginary ones.

The learning of the Island of the Lost Illusions is that, face to the unexpected, we can rely on our resources of intuition and improvisation,

Emotions	Resources
• Feeling out of place	• Coping strategies
• Restlessnes	• Instincts
• Confusion	• Intuition
• Panic, anguish	• Improvisation

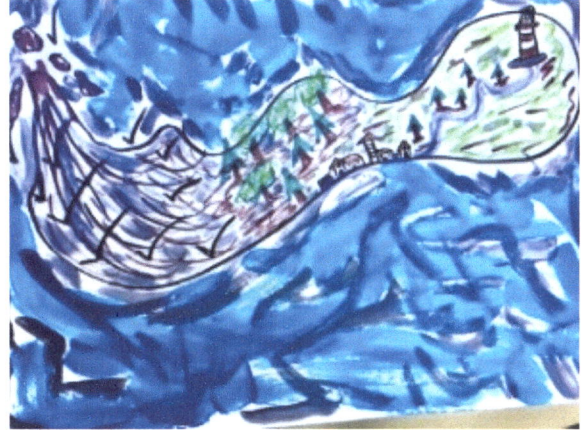

Fig. 7.3 SDM 2: Bewilderment

7.3.3   The Island of the Brave New World

See Fig. 7.4.

On the third SDM we realized how much we had missed the pleasure of the aimless wandering around in the streets of the city, driven by the curiosity to explore in an open landscape and by the desire to get out of the comfort zone of home that had gradually turned into a prison.

In the Island of the Brave New World we enter an unfamiliar landscape, with no known landmarks, in which the first striking evidence is that nothing is the same as it was before. At first we are gripped by anxiety, which is soon replaced by a feeling of nostalgia for the old, well known, idealized world we have left behind, which seems unattainable now.

Suddenly however another transformation occurs, what we felt before as a tension of opposite feelings that kept us from moving forward turned into a challenge, pushed by the curiosity to find out what is around the corner.

We took courage, telling ourselves that the journey may be fun after all. We met strange characters on the way, but they proved at the end to be the helpers we needed so much to adjust survive in the new world.

The most precious treasure of this island was therefore the discovery of inner resources of courage, playfulness, intuition, imagination, together with the trust in others, that can be looked at as helpers instead of enemies.

Emotions	Resources
• Anxiety	• Flanerie
• Longing	• Playfulness
• Distortion of reality	• Fantasy
• Astonishment	• Courage

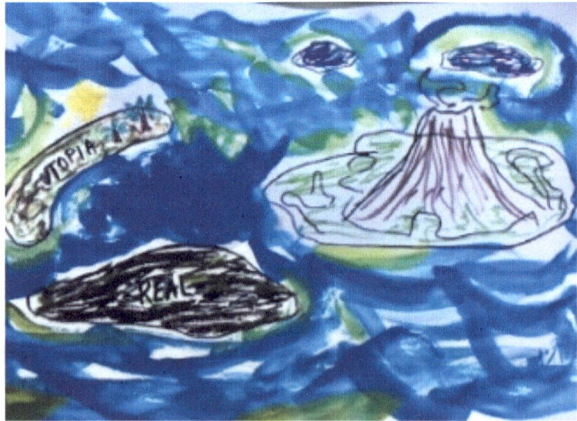

Fig. 7.4 SDM 3: Wandering Around, Flanerie

7.3.4   The Island of the Magical Thinking

See Fig. 7.5.

At the end of the journey, in the fourth SDM, the Island of Magical Thinking appears, at first glance, as a beautiful exciting world, in which it is possible to indulge to the pleasures of senses, rediscovering emotions we had not been accustomed to for long. The intensity of the colors, the depth of sensations, the lightness of the air, were wonderfully intoxicating. The power of desires makes us feel invincible, wondering to have fantastic superpowers. We felt powerful and energized by the new life.

But could we really trust the newfound arousing pleasures? Or could those pleasurable feelings conceal an ego inflation?

The newly rediscovered excitement of all senses may hide hallucination, the sexual arousal may cover anger and aggression, behind the fantasies of being empowered and invincible may lurk the fear of being harmless. Hallucination is the domain of the magical thinking, a kind of anti-thinking based on fantasies of omnipotence that replace the actual reality with an invented one, because we are unable to endure the split between the inner and the outer world. Hallucination is a trap in which we could once again being caught, a field of missed opportunities in which no transformation happens.

The last island represents therefore, at the same time, a wish and a warning.

In the island of Magical Thinking we discover the need for a reflexive stance, the possibility of activating a double gaze, a sight which is turned partly outward and partly inward. To escape the danger of a regression toward the traumatic situation of the beginning, we should allow ourselves the long time of introspection, in a dialogue with our internal characters, shadows, fears.

Rebirth, the coming to a new life, requires to activate an "inner gaze", which is both an inward and an outward gaze, a process of self-discovery that renews our ties with the world.

Fig. 7.5 SDM 4: Return

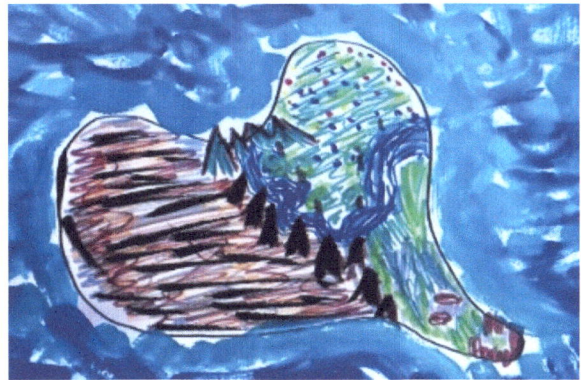

The last island tells us that the journey is not over, that it has just begun, inviting us to experience the thrill of the new possible discoveries.

Emotions	Resources
• Excitement	• Pleasure, sensoriality
• Aggression	• Inner sight
• Paranoia	• Rebirth
• Hallucination	• Repair

7.4   The New Argonauts

> This mood makes itself felt everywhere, politically, socially, and philosophically. We are living in what the Greeks called the Kairos - the right time - for a "metamorphosis of the gods", i.e. of the fundamental principles and symbols. (C.G. Jung [6], The Undiscovered Self)

The story of the extraordinary voyage of the Argonauts in search of the Golden Fleece was the starting point of our story and is also our point of arrival. Since the beginning of our journey, in fact, we felt the myth of the Argonauts could have been a beautiful metaphor for the urgency of a departure. As modern Argonauts, we set out on a journey toward an uncertain destination, moved by the common feeling that the pandemic had left us no choice, but could have been an opportunity to challenge our own destiny. The urge to find new points of reference in a complex reality, to draw new maps to explore an unfamiliar territory, surfaced from the dark shadows that threatened the future and required to deploy new energies to cope with change.

The expedition of the Argonauts in search of the Golden Fleece was described by Apollonio Rodio in his poem Le Argonautiche, one of the most fascinating myths of antiquity. Its unfolding celebrates not only the feat of a single hero, but rather tells of a community of purpose, when all the most extraordinary characters of ancient Greece gathered around a hero by chance, Jason, all of them driven more by the desire to undertake the journey than by the need to accomplish the deed.

Perhaps this is the true meaning behind the Argonauts' expedition, an encouragement to make the most of the time we are given, as the heroes and fellow travelers did at their time, pursuing a fate that is never just an individual destiny, but is a mutual enterprise guided by destiny.

As Roberto Calasso wrote:

> The appearance of the heroes covers a very short period in the history of Greece. They knew each other, or had listened to stories about the others from those who had known them. Like links on a bracelet, the cycle of Crete, the cycle of the Argonauts, the cycle of Thebes, the cycle of Troy succeeded. And everything burns out in a few years…. The heroes sealed the significant events and disappeared. Speed was part of their essence. It is as if the Greeks had wanted to concentrate in a minimum segment of time all the stories whose consequences they would have lived afterwards. [7, p. 126]

Human history has always needed heroes, as well as myths and stories to tell the tale of their deeds.

Our contemporary society has no longer myths—the last one, the American Dream, is now showing clear signs of fatigue—and it is increasingly evident that we miss them badly. Just as we miss the "heroic" enterprises, capable of linking thought and action, to restore sense of challenge that can guide us toward the future.

Blessed are those peoples who have no need of heroes, goes a famous quote by Bertolt Brecht, which I never subscribed. On the contrary, we believe that today more than ever we need to recover a "heroic feeling" that could allow us to intertwine individual destinies and collective stories, rediscovering the sense of a common becoming, as well as the will and the capacity to act in a conscious and responsible manner.

The Journey of Dreams during the pandemic was for us an important push in this direction, full of enlightening insights that make us look forward to future challenges. This is therefore not the end of the story, but the beginning of a new adventure in which we hope to engage soon again with other fellow travelers.

References

1. Mapelli B. Nuove intimità. In: Strategie affettive e comunitarie nel pluralismo contemporaneo. Torino: Rosemberg e Sellier; 2018.
2. Castiglioni M. Pedagogia dei transiti nell'età adulta. Pisa: Edizioni ETS; 2021.
3. Heiddeger M. Sentieri interrotti. Firenze. La Nuova Italia; 1968.
4. Amicucci F. Apprendere nell'infosfera. Milano: Franco Angeli; 2022.
5. Borgna E. In dialogo con la solitudine. Torino: Einaudi; 2021.
6. Jung CG. The undiscovered self. Routledge, NY: Paperback; 2013.
7. Calasso R. Le nozze di Cadmo e Armonia. Adelphi; 1988.
8. Rodio A. Le Argonautiche. Milano: BUR-Rizzoli Libri; 1986.

Glossary

Active Imagination Conceived by Jung in the Red Book as an imaginative process, Active Imagination takes the dreams in a "prospective" way, amplifying and visualizing them through symbols, images, and narratives in order to bridge the conscious ego with the unconscious contents. In a therapeutic process Active Imagination builds on the less controlled activities of the mind like daydreaming, spontaneous fantasies, reveries, obsessive thinking, to activate the creative parts of the self via imagination and fantasy.

Amplification Amplification is a part of Jung's method of interpretation of clinical and cultural material, especially dreams. Involves the use of mythic, historical, and cultural parallels in order to clarify, make more ample, and, so to speak, turn up the volume on materials that may be obscure, thin, and difficult to attend to (see Andrew Samuels). Amplification is also a means of exploring the Jungian concept of the collective unconscious, whose early understanding was that it consisted of primordial images (the archetypes) that were, to a large degree, consistent across cultures and historical epochs.

Analytical Psychology Analytical Psychology or Complex Psychology is a term created by the Swiss Psychiatrist C.G.Jung to distinguish his analytical method from Freud's psychoanalysis. Among the most widely used concepts specific to Analytical Psychology are archetypes, the collective unconscious, complexes, extraversion and introversion, psychological types, individuation, and the Self. The foundation of Analytical Psychology and its development as the study and practice of psychology in connection with other human sciences and disciplines can be found in Jung's monumental opus, the Collected Works, written over 60 years of his lifetime.

Archetype Archetypes are a concept from Jungian's Analytical Psychology that refer to universal, inherited ideas, pattern of thoughts, or images that are present in the collective unconscious of all human beings. The psychic counterpart of instincts, archetypes are thought to be the basis of many of the common themes and symbols that appear in stories, myths, and dreams across different cultures and societies. Some examples of archetypes include the Great Mother, the Child, the Shadow, the Trickster, the Hero, the Old Wise Man, among others.

Free Associations Basic process of psychoanalysis and psychodynamic psychotherapy in which the patient is encouraged to verbalize without censorship or selection whatever thoughts come to mind, no matter how embarrassing, illogical, or irrelevant they may be. The object is to allow unconscious material, such as inhibited thoughts and emotions, traumatic experiences, or threatening impulses, to come to the surface, where they can help the patient to discharge some of the feelings that have given this material excessive control over him or her.

Habitat It is the set of dream images expressed in the dreams for each Social Dreaming session, enclosed in a common frame. The word Habitat refers to the inner landscape, revealed by the social dreams, which includes dialogue with the outer context. The concept of Habitat that we have used in this manuscript is an attempt to capture the dynamic between the external and internal worlds during each Social Dreaming matrix.

Individual and Collective Unconscious The term collective unconscious was firstly introduced by C.G. Jung to describe the unconscious part of the mind containing memories and impulses of which the individual is not aware, which are common to mankind as a whole and originate in the inherited structure of the brain. The collective unconscious is distinct from the Freudian personal unconscious, which arises from the experience of the individual and contains mainly repressed sexual impulses and desires. According to Jung, archetypes are the contents of the collective unconscious as universal primordial images and ideas common to the mankind; they can be revealed through the analysis of dreams as images and patterns that strongly influence individual behaviors.

Initiation Initiation is the set of rites and ceremonies that sanction the passage of an individual as a member of a group from one status to another. The life of individuals is made of many different phases: we grow up from childhood to adulthood to the old age; we fell in love, get married and separate, we go through births and deaths of beloved ones; we move, change jobs and countries, meet some new people and leave some others behind. Initiation implies a change of status and a new beginning; it is a "moments of passage" in life and a precious occasion for a better understanding of the changes in and around us, which can lead to new surprising discoveries, increasing the self-awareness of inner potentialities. But unlike in the past, all these stages of life are today mostly experienced in solitude, often perceived as existential crisis bringing anxiety and uncertainty about the future, questioning ones identity, requiring a radical change of attitudes and behaviors.

Listening Post Listening Posts are regular meetings that take a "snapshot" of society at a particular moment in time. A methodology developed by OPUS—The Organisation for the Promotion of Social Understanding in Society (https://www.opus.org.uk/listening-posts/), LP explores the idea that a small group, when studying the behavior of the wider social system that is society, will unconsciously express some of the characteristics of society and that these are discernible from the themes and patterns emerging from the discussion. Since they originated in 1975, Listening Posts have been developed and standardized by OPUS. The current format of the International Listening Post Project was adopted in 2000 and is now convened on an annual basis, in January of each year, in around thirty countries under the guidance and coordination of OPUS. These are all presented in a common format as a Global Report. This research now has several years of Global Reports to compare and is generating valuable data that is increasing in relevance as the effects of globalization are felt throughout the world.

Matrix The current definition of matrix, taken from the Encyclopedia Britannica, is "a rectangular arrangement of a collection of numbers into a fixed number of rows and columns" that constitutes the underlying structure of reality. However, matrix in also an ambiguous term that can have different opposing meanings. Here it's used in its literal meaning of womb, a generative space in which something new can happen, a definition Gordon Lawrence derived from S.H. Foulkes.

Myth Myth, from the Greek word Mythos, equal to word, discourse, has the meaning of an imaginary narrative that refers to the idealized past of a community, its origins and institutions, and features heroes and deities. Jungian Analytical Psychology considers myths to be collective manifestations of the human mind whose unconscious tendencies they reveal.

Narrative Medicine (NM) or Narrative-Based Medicine (NNM) Narrative-Based Medicine (EBM) is a new medical paradigm born at the beginning of the 1990s, which enhances the use of disease stories and promotes the development of an approach to humanization of care in the practice of medicine. Narrative medicine is part of the medical humanities, or the humanities applied to the field of health, illness, and treatment. Its roots can be found in art whenever through figurative and literary works the theme of health and illness has been given space.

RÊVERIE The word "rêverie," imported from French, is commonly used like daydreaming and fantastic thinking, in its dual meaning of the one who indulges in reveries and the expression of the reverie. The British psychoanalyst Wilfred Bion was the first to give to the concept of reverie a new specific psychoanalytic meaning: in his famous book *Learning from Experience*, reverie indicates the mother's ability to hold the emotional and sensory impressions of the infant and process them in a form that the infant's psyche can reintroject and assimilate. The Bionian theory of thought thus hypothesizes that experience cannot become thinkable, either consciously or unconsciously, unless it is transformed into elementary representations (the alpha elements) by the work of a psychic function called at first alpha dream work and later alpha function.

Ritual A ritual or rite means a set of repetitive behaviors consisting of actions, words, and gestures endowed with symbolic value, the meaning of which is understandable to the community people belong to or at least some of the participants in the ritual. Performing or adhering to a ritual thus means being part of an established order of a religious character or belonging to a community whose rules and traditions are shared. The concept of "mystical participation" that Jung takes from the French anthropologist Lucien Levy Bruhl indicates the sense of unity and common feeling that participating in a ritual arouses.

Semiotic Semiotics is defined as the general science of signs, their production, transmission and interpretation, or the ways in which something is communicated and signified, or an otherwise symbolic object is produced. The term semiotic was first used in the early 1900s to denote an autonomous discipline that had as its object the functioning of sign systems, whether natural or artificial.

Semiotic Square One of the most relevant figures in the semiotic structure of discourse, introduced by Algirdas Greimas to indicate the fundamental values underlying and the contrasts that define the nature of their relationships within a narrative, giving movement to the story. The representation of these elements is done through a graphic scheme, the so-called "semiotic square."

Setting Setting, from the English word to set which means to arrange and to establish, can be defined in clinical psychology as the set of conditions that delimit, accommodate, and support the relationship between the therapist and the patient. Defining the setting for the psychologist means delimiting the boundaries within which he or she constructs a physical and mental space for the client. The ways of conceiving, organizing, and using the setting in psychological-clinical intervention are closely intertwined with the theoretical approach, the methodologies that the clinician uses in his work. The psychodynamic approach recognizes the value of the processes of unconscious symbolization and operational categorization of reality as a function of the relationship with the other within a peculiar institutional context of reference by considering the intertwining of the affective, cognitive, social, and institutional dimensions in psychological-clinical intervention.

Social Dreaming Social Dreaming is a way of working with dreams where the focus is on the dream and not the dreamer. A methodology created by the psychoanalyst Gordon Lawrence at the end of the 70s, Social Dreaming grounds on the ancient technique of the social meaning of dreams. Dreaming has always been used by many cultures in the world, from the native Americans, Africans, Australians, to the ancient Greeks, Egyptians, Chinese, as a prominent way to capture thinking about the past and learning about the present, while guiding people toward the future. Social Dreaming builds on this legacy to bring new thinking and meaning to the contemporary society in which we live and work. Dreams are images of our inner emotions, linking us with a collective whole we can share and expand. When safely shared and worked with, dreams offer understanding and new learning, becoming a powerful source of creativity. Social Dreaming is used in organizations, groups, associations, communities, projects, events, conferences, or stand-alone forums for discovering the communal meaning in our dreams. Opening the mind to dreams by sharing them with others generates new thinking, makes us discover new knowledge, and opens up our mind to different perspectives. Social Dreaming is a pleasurable and revealing experience where participants learn to think divergently, breaking from the more typical goal-orientation discourse.

Social Dreaming Matrix Key to a Social Dreaming event is the "matrix," a place where we come together to share and explore our dreams: a "hosted" experience in which we share dreams, associate to dreams, derive from them collective meanings, develop new creative thoughts. The associative process of the matrix allows for the open, non-judgmental expression of thoughts, allowing participants to foster free thinking and social interaction to co-create new meaning.

Symbol The word symbol comes from the Greek word "symballein," which means to throw together, to join together. A symbol is composed of something visible, the objects we perceive in reality, and something invisible, the hidden ideal surface of reality. This means that everything we experience in the world has a deeper meaning, refers to something profound. C.G. Jung connects the formation of symbols with the tension of opposites: in his view, human life in general is constituted in a symbolic way, and whatever we experience, represent, and shape also refers to an unconscious background, which is expressed in these symbols. The resulting "transcendent function" consists of conveying symbolic conscious and unconscious contents.

Synchronicity Referred to the subjective experience of coincidences between events in one's mind and the outside world that may be causally unrelated to each other and yet perceived as having unknown connections, synchronicity was firstly introduced in psychology by C.G. Jung as key concept of his vision of the world and of the relationship between psyche and matter. Synchronicity was defined by Jung as an acausal connecting principle, whereby internal, psychological events are linked to external world events by meaningful coincidences rather than causal chains. Strongly influenced by the Chinese Taoist Philosophy, synchronicity is largely used in modern physics to explain the origin of the universe, and was the object of a larger cosmological vision achieved by Jung's collaboration with the famous Nobel Laureate physicist Wolfgang Pauli. Their correspondence holds many keys to the evolution of the hypothesis as marriage of physics and psychology.

Transitional Space The concept of transitional space and transitional object was firstly introduced by the British psychoanalyst Donald Winnicott. It originates in that phase of an infant's development when inner and outer reality begin to become apparent. They are at once "me" and "not-me," and are transitional in that they facilitate the transition from the omnipotence of the tiny baby for whom external objects have not yet separated out, to the capacity to relate to "objectively perceived" objects. Winnicott used the term transitional to describe the "intermediate" or "third area," where fantasy and reality overlap, and that creativity, including the basis for adult cultural life, and play originate. Winnicott compared this with the therapeutic situation, where the worlds of the patient and analyst overlap, echoing Freud's concept of the analytic playground.

GPSR Compliance

The European Union's (EU) General Product Safety Regulation (GPSR) is a set of rules that requires consumer products to be safe and our obligations to ensure this.

If you have any concerns about our products, you can contact us on ProductSafety@springernature.com

In case Publisher is established outside the EU, the EU authorized representative is:

Springer Nature Customer Service Center GmbH
Europaplatz 3
69115 Heidelberg, Germany

The manufacturer's authorised representative in the EU is Springer
Nature Customer Service Centre GmbH, Europaplatz 3, 69115 Heidelberg,
Germany. If you have any concerns regarding our products, please
contact ProductSafety@springernature.com

Printed and bound by CPI Group (UK) Ltd, Croydon, CR0 4YY
30/04/2026
02100216-0003